IF THEY COULD ONLY HEAR ME

ISBN: 1-4196-2245-5

Fist Edition 2005

Preface

This is a book about unusual heroes. The heroes in this book are usually thought of as victims. But these are heroes who refused to be considered victims in life; and they are heroes who would not want to be remembered as victims after their passing. What follows, we sincerely hope, is a celebration of their lives and a tribute to the contribution each has made in furthering the battle to discover the causes and, one day soon, the cure that will ultimately eradicate the medical scourge known as Lou Gehrig's disease.

Lou Gehrig's disease, or amyotrophic lateral sclerosis (ALS), is a progressive, neuromuscular disease with no known cause or cure. It is characterized by a degeneration of nerve cells in the brain and spinal cord, ones that control muscle movement. These nerve cells begin to wither and die, leading to an unrelenting weakening of muscles throughout the body. As the disease progresses, total paralysis and the inability to speak or swallow result. The mind and senses remain intact and unaffected, a tormenting daily reminder to the victim of all that has been lost. Death generally follows in three-to-five years.

Relatively little known for decades, and particularly difficult to diagnose as well, ALS has, tragically, recently experienced a surge in cases identified. Considering how rare occurrences of ALS affliction once were, some medical experts are calling the present rate of diagnosed cases "an epidemic." Today, in the United States alone, there are more than 30,000 known cases.

"If They Could Only Hear Me" is an attempt to give a voice to a variety of different perspectives about this insidious disease. Included in these pages are accounts from those afflicted themselves, husbands and wives of those afflicted, children of the afflicted, and others who would surely consider themselves extended family members, such as close friends and respectful professional peers. Even included are doctors and care-givers, several of whom saw relationships evolve into something far more intimate, far more respectful and even loving, than usual practitioner-patient relationships. Indeed, a sense of "family" seems pervasive.

And that idea of "family" would be wholly fitting: For the concrete connection between all the stories contained within would be the connection to the Angel Fund, a research fund seeking to find causes and, ultimately, a cure for ALS. Established at Mass General Hospital in Boston in the late 1990s, the fund supports the research work of Dr. Robert Brown.

Seeing the bonds that grew from so many individuals attracted to join and whole-heartedly support the work of the Angel Fund, Paul DelVecchio, the fund's executive director, had the inspiration, during the summer of 2004, to find a way to celebrate heroes, celebrate families, and, indeed, celebrate voices that deserved to be heard!

We are grateful to all those members of the Angel Fund "family" who accepted our blanket invitation to write their stories and share them. These are their stories, so they will be heard and remembered, in the special way each deserves.

Ed Rice
Editor

Table of Contents

1.   Craig Boyce on FREDERICK BOYCE......................................1

2.   Lauren Bradbury on DAVID A. ODAMS........................5

3.   Dr. Robert H. Brown on GINNY DelVECCHIO.................9

4.   Bill and Kay Byers on WILLIE BYERS......................11

6.   Barry Chait on SCOTT CARLSON.............................13

7.   Paul DelVecchio...17

8.   Todd DelVecchio on GINNY DelVECCHIO..................19

9.   Kim DiRocco on WILLIE BYERS..............................23

10. Sal Falzone on GINNY DelVECCHIO........................27

11. Anne Fucillo on GINNY DelVECCHIO......................29

12. Roberta "Bobbi" Gibb on BUCK............................31

13. Ann Hadley...41

14. Jillian Hensley on SCOTT CARLSON......................43

15. Tracy Hill on SHARON TIMLIN.............................47

16. Drew Hoffman...49

17. Richard Kennedy on CHRISTOPHER and JIMMY KENNEDY......51

18. Dr. Thomas Kwiatkowski, Jr...............................55

19. GEORGE MAZAREAS..57

20. Maureen Neil on JIMMIE NEIL.............................59

21. Derek Pearson poem on DAVID ODAMS....................63

22. Ed Rice on RICHARD KISONAK and GINNY DelVECCHIO......65

23. Debra Rohan on KAY SANDERS............................73

24. Ron Sanders on KAY SANDERS.............................77

25. Irene Scaturro on FRANK SCATURRO and G. DelVECCHIO......79

26. Jane Schulte on SHARON TIMLIN.........................83

27. Jan Serieka poem on GINNY DelVECCHIO..................85

28. H. S. Sherrill..87

29. Mike Timlin on SHARON TIMLIN..........................91

30. Mark Zullo on MARILYN ZULLO...........................93

By Craig Boyce

Sadly, I was introduced to the horrific disease called ALS just over 10 years ago. I'd spent much of my senior year in college trying to understand what was ailing my father. We didn't know what was causing his speech to be slurred, why his hands were growing so frail. The heartbreaking news was delivered the day after I graduated from Princeton. My celebratory moment atop one of life's pinnacles was cut short by the medical declaration that my father was sentenced to a life with this terrible disease.

Convinced there must be something I could do to stop my father's ALS, I spent the following summer performing research and development work at Merck, by day, and did ALS research in the library, by night. The more I learned about the disease, the more troubled I became: There was a 3-5 year life expectancy, and no known cause or cure. It featured a slow and steady deterioration of nerve cells, creating muscle atrophy and, ultimately, paralysis. All the while the mind remained intact. It seemed so cruel that I was left with only one question: Why?

During the fall of 1994, I made my way to Boston for graduate school at MIT, with the hope of finding a research project searching for a cure for ALS. After a year and one- half, I was left frustrated by the lack of projects I found focused on ALS. Further, I was unable to dedicate myself to detailed, tangential research while I worried about my family's financial and emotional health. So I left the world of academia for business. Underlying my career change was a conviction that I would be more productive raising money for ALS research, than performing it. At the same time, I wanted to ensure that neither my college-aged brother's education, nor my 13-year-old brother's life would be interrupted or uprooted by financial uncertainty.

Throughout the three-plus years that my father struggled with the disease, rarely did I see him without a smile. I attribute this to my mother's fortitude and her relentless efforts as a caretaker. Despite his horrible predicament, my father found daily joy in the little things in life, which allowed him to view his circumstances as tolerable. From the fall of 1994 until my father's death in February of 1997, I made many trips from Boston to New Jersey in order to enjoy my father's company for as much and as long as possible, as well as to support my family.

During the ordeal, I, too, came to savor the "little things" more than ever before – enjoying a collective family laugh watching "Seinfeld," cheering the Yankees to a World Series victory, exchanging e-mails with thoughts on life and career paths with my father, gathering for family dinners, and even providing my father food through a feeding tube. Each activity provided a certain, special bond.

After my father passed away, a huge void emerged that I longed to fill. My goal was to find some way to support others who were suffering from ALS, as a way to memorialize my father. I saw such an effort as a path to self-healing. I continued to try to make it back to New Jersey as often as possible to support my mother and my youngest brother. And I became a volunteer with the Massachusetts Chapter of the national ALS association, helping to raise money at first through annual ALS walks. I then joined that chapter's board and spent five years assisting the development and growth of the organization. During that time we tripled its budget and financial resources, further developing its patient services programs and expanding its patient reach.

Having been inspired by Dr. Robert Brown's research developments and the refreshing focus he and his associates share in seeking to find a cure for ALS, I joined the board of The Angel Fund in 2003.

The one constant throughout my service over the last eight years has been my dedication to raising money and awareness through an annual walk for ALS; for the past two years, I have participated in The Angel Fund's Walk of Hope. In total, I have now raised in excess of $250,000 for a cause that has been dedicated to funding patient services and funding research to find a cure. In addition to raising money for such a worthy cause, I have found that this entire experience has enriched my life through the many wonderful people that I have met in the ALS community and Angel Fund family. Also, through these opportunities I have participated in events that have afforded me the chance to gather with my family and friends for a day of hope and a day of remembrance… remembrance of an amazing father, Frederick Boyce, who inspired it all.

Along the way, many people have assisted with my efforts and contributed to the achievements in more ways than imaginable. Many thanks and much gratitude go to the following: To my family, without whom none of this would be possible. They include: my loving wife, Maureen; my mom, Margaret; two brothers, Eric and John; sister, Carrie; and all my extended family, including grandparents, in-laws, aunts and uncles.

Also, thanks to Bain Capital, my colleagues and friends, as well as all who have generously supported my fund-raising efforts – especially Josh Bekenstein, whose generosity has helped enable me to raise sizeable sums of money for ALS .

Additionally, "Thank You" to all my fellow current and former board members on both The Angel Fund and ALS Association-Massachusetts Chapter, who have worked tirelessly in the fight against ALS.

Finally, I wish to express my gratitude to all the patients, caregivers and members of the ALS community who keep a smile while fighting this horrible disease. There is hope through Dr. Brown's research.

By Lauren Bradbury

(Editor's note: Asked to write about her husband, David A. Odams, for this book, his widow, Linda commented: "…I gave much thought to what to write. Each time I sat down I couldn't put into words our story. Maybe it's too soon; maybe I'll never be able to put into words the story of David Alden Odams. David had just turned 34 years old in November of 1997 when he was diagnosed with Lou Gehrig's disease; our children were just 5, 3 and 1 years old. We were devastated. Our friends and family all shared in our heartbreak as we watched our beautiful, strong, loving man lose so much. Thanks to our friend Mary Hartley, who started an Angel Fund golf tournament seven years ago, we found strength in all the support we received from our family, friends and community. David was never alone. The golf tournament has now become one day out of the year that our children and I can truly celebrate Dave and seeing all the people who cared for their father is such a gift for our children…I would like to share a letter that I think shares a touch of David.")

Dear David, Kaitlyn & Billy:

Shortly after your daddy passed away, your mom asked if I could write a little something about him that you kids would be able to read when you got older. She wanted to make sure that you would always remember what a great guy he was, and how much he was involved in research and fund-raising to help find a cure for ALS. It has taken me a while to be able to sit and write this, but with the holiday season approaching I find myself thinking about you and your mom, and I know that this is going to be a very difficult time for all of you.

I am a nurse at Mass General Hospital. All of my patients have ALS, and they are all wonderful people with great families. As much as I care for all of my patients, your dad was my favorite. Nurses are not supposed to have favorites, but there was just something about your dad…his personality, his sense of humor, his generosity, the way his eyes lit up when he talked about his wife and children.

Your dad was in one of our clinical trials to test a drug for ALS. He had a pump put in his belly and every day the pump would give him medicine that we hoped would slow down the ALS. He came to Mass General Hospital every month for almost two years, and never once did he ever complain about all the tests, blood draws, and pump refills that we had to do. I looked forward to his visits, and I would always make sure he was the only patient scheduled on the day he was coming in so I would have plenty of time just to hang out with him.

Not once did he ever tell me that he didn't feel good, even when I could tell that he was having a bad day. He was strong and brave and courageous; he was a true hero. ALS may have taken control of his muscles, but it never took his spirit.

He always wanted to know how I was, and what was going on in my life. One day your dad came in for an appointment and it was snowing really hard outside. He was here with his friends, CJ and Ray, and we were talking about the weather. I told your dad I wasn't looking forward to going home that night and shoveling my driveway. He asked for my address and told me he would come by and plow with one of his trucks. (It didn't matter that I live almost one and one-half hours from Plainville, and at this point your dad couldn't drive anymore – he was going to take a ride with one of his buddies and plow my driveway!)

At that point we had our first "argument" – I wouldn't give him my address! I told him Linda would kill me if he was out driving around in a blizzard. We had a really good laugh that day. That's the kind of guy he was…if I had given him my address he would have been there. He always put everyone else before himself. He was totally selfless with a heart of gold. He was more than a patient; he was my friend. I learned so much from him.

When your dad died my heart broke. It is so hard to understand why someone so young and full of life has to be taken from us so soon. I come to work every day and hope that we will come one step closer to finding a cure for ALS so no more wives will lose a wonderful husband and no more children will have to grow up without their daddy. Money that your dad raised at his golf tournaments is helping us find that cure.

There are no words that can describe the love that your dad had for you and your mom. You were his whole world, and I hope that you never forget that. Just the mention of your names brought a huge smile to his face – he was so proud of all of you.

As the holidays approach, and I think about Thanksgiving and Christmas, I realize that your dad was truly a gift and I am blessed to have known him. The world would be such a better place I there were more guys like him. I will never forget your dad, and I hope that your memories of him will help you through the tough times.

God was looking for an angel on March 3, 2002, and your dad volunteered, because that's the kind of guy he was.

You are always in my thoughts.

By Robert H. Brown, Jr.

Ginny and Paul DelVecchio are two extraordinary and unforgettable people. I first met Ginny and Paul at a devastating time in their lives, when Ginny's mother and brother had been afflicted by ALS.

Remarkable from the start was the commitment Paul and Ginny demonstrated to finding a cure for this terrible disease. Their response to the double tragedy in the family was to establish the first Massachusetts chapter of the ALS Association, for which they labored intensively and successfully. We met on many occasions during those years, typically at patient and caregiver meetings.

Ginny's warmth, kindness and helpfulness to people newly diagnosed with ALS made her the proverbial pillar of strength; she gave reassurance and support to all, including caregivers and doctors, as well as her friends with ALS and their families. Having lived the tragedy of seeing two close family members succumb to ALS, she worked ceaselessly to support efforts to cure the disease, in the hope that no one would ever suffer the ALS scourge as she had.

It was therefore almost unbearable to receive an urgent phone call one afternoon from Ginny who was recovering from an upper respiratory infection and congestion when she rather abruptly developed slurring of speech. Paul, Ginny and I met immediately to assess the situation. No effort was spared in the attempt to discern a treatable cause for the speech problem. Yet, as each week passed, our certainty that this was ALS grew, as test after test, and progressive slurring of speech, foreclosed all other possibilities. When the diagnosis became inevitable, Ginny and Paul faced her situation with characteristic strength and determination.

Ginny continued to work as a school teacher for months, using first a cane and then teaching from her wheelchair. In the face of progressive weakness, she was a picture of strength and dignity to her students, illuminating by her own example, the meaning of courage. When strength of breathing and moving ebbed to the danger point, Ginny elected to go on a respirator, convinced that she would still be able to work with Paul to wage their continuing battle against ALS.

At about that point, when many others might have gently backed away from the struggle, Ginny and Paul opted to increase their efforts in the ALS battle. With family members and friends, they founded the Angel Fund as a vehicle to intensify and focus their efforts. Although her limbs no longer moved, and her speech failed, Ginny continued to radiate, through her eyes, the perceptive caring that was her signature and to motivate everyone she knew to join her struggle.

Many stirring examples come immediately to mind, especially the extraordinary efforts of Ed Rice, who ran daily back-to-back marathons in his own one-man Massachusetts challenge, running across the state to raise funds for Ginny and the Angel Fund.

In those early days, and indeed ceaselessly since, Paul was an irrepressible force for the fund, establishing contacts and raising funds with passion.

As weeks of total paralysis became months, and then years, Ginny experienced increasing respiratory infections and more numerous hospital visits. At the same time, her ability to communicate faltered as the movements of those remarkable eyes slowed and then ceased altogether. Quietly but resolutely, she decided that the end had come. We gathered at her bedside one extraordinary afternoon to bid her farewell and bon voyage.

Others will describe more eloquently the many dimensions of Ginny's legacy. It extends across a wide domain of family, students and friends. For all of us whose lives she touched, Ginny's vision and goodness are still with us. For those of us in ALS research, both Ginny and Paul remain a constant inspiration.

In only five years, the Angel Fund has had an unmistakable impact on ALS research, funding numerous ALS scientists from the U.S. and abroad, equipping the laboratory at the Massachusetts General Hospital for a new, state-of-the art genetics program, and facilitating study of novel approaches to ALS treatment.

There is little doubt that Ginny's dream will be realized in the foreseeable future – that effective therapy will guarantee that no one will suffer from ALS as Ginny did. When that day arrives, Ginny's legacy will be fulfilled.

By Bill and Kay Byers

As our son, Willie, was suffering the effects of ALS, an angel of mercy visited him. That angel was Kim DiRocco.

Willie, who had known Kim since their childhood days, was a friend of Kim's husband, Todd. At Todd's urging, Kim became involved in Willie's care, on a strictly volunteer basis, and began twice-weekly visits to perform respiratory therapy to aid Willie's breathing. As the disease progressed Kim was available to our family whenever she was needed and frequently visited just to see if she could be of help in any way.

On numerous occasions, when hospitalization was required, Kim would be at the hospital along with members of our family, providing comfort and support. As things got worse Kim spent more and more time at Willie's house, even spending her days off from her job at Lowell General Hospital. In order to give Willie's wife, Camille, a much needed break, Kim stayed over on weekends so that Camille could get away from the stress for a couple of days.

So intense and loving was her support it was only fitting that Kim was present when the end came on April 13, 2000.

After Willie's passing, Kim has remained in close contact with our family, providing love and friendship in her very special way.

Kim started a golf tournament in Willie's name and became involved in the Angel Fund to support others who suffer from ALS. That golf tournament continues today and recognizes many people who have suffered from ALS. Our family provides financial and operational support in the running of that very successful charitable event.

Kim DiRocco has been a rock of strength during a very stressful time for our family. There are not enough words in the dictionary to describe how we feel about Kim and the contributions that she has made. Loving, sincere, respectful of our privacy and professional in her dealings with a delicate situation are only a few of the attributes that come to mind.

Thank you, Kim, for all that you have done and continue to do for us.

We love you.

By Barry N. Chait

If they could only hear me? But I honestly believe they can. Eleven years ago I was fortunate enough to be going to a Red Sox game and my friend, Dennis Tetreault, convinced me to run the Boston Marathon for the American Liver Foundation. That day will live in "infamy" for me...because that day changed my whole life. Now I have completed 10 Boston Marathons, raising money for the American Liver Foundation and the Angel Fund.

Why do I run? Because I am fortunate enough to be healthy and want to give back to the community. I want to do something good for others.

The journey to the Angel Fund traveled through the Thursday night charity program runs, first to the Elliot Lounge, and then to Crossroads Pub. During marathon training season, we have met at one of the above mentioned bars and traveled to the Woodland T-stop to run the last nine miles of the Boston Marathon course.

Being one of the slower runners, I would be in the back of the pack and every Thursday night I would see the members of Team Psycho go running past me and hear someone yell the same encouragement to me, "Go, Liver Guy!" Several times I asked my friend, Matt Bergin, who that was, and he'd tell me: "Scott Carlson...You know who he is; he runs on New Year's Day with us." I still wasn't positive about the name, but there was that same voice, Thursday after Thursday. I accepted that Matt was right.

Then one day my friends Meg Reynolds and Skip McKee told me that Scott had ALS...Lou Gehrig's disease. Being an avid baseball fan I could only think of the film "Pride of the Yankees," and what a terrible disease ALS is. During this period I found out that my friends Jake and Rat Kennedy's brother had ALS, and that their father had also had the disease and died of it. Thinking of how terrible this all was, I was determined that we must do something. Anything.

During this period I began talking to the Harpoon Brewery about sponsoring a charity road race. Once I convinced them that it was a good business decision and great for the community, we had to decide what charity to which we should donate the proceeds. Liver Foundation? Dana Farber? No...the truly correct charity here was the Angel Fund. Harpoon was already sponsoring Team Psycho – the team to which Scott Carlson proudly belonged – and we learned that one of the founders of Harpoon had died of ALS. The message was all too clear. We could hear them then.

A committee was pulled together and, today, the race has become one of the most successful runs in the Boston area. Still, I believe the potential is there for the run to do even more – to raise substantial sums of money for ALS research and the Angel Fund, to bring more good will for the Angel Fund, and to help make more people aware of this horrendous disease. Without our great race committee and the commitment from Harpoon Brewery, and our burning desire to help find a cure for ALS, this would be just another road race. We believe in the cause and the committee members all believe that we are just so fortunate to be healthy and to be able to give something back.

It was at the first annual Harpoon 5-Miler to benefit the Angel Fund that Scott Carlson's wife, Hillary, said: "Barry, Scott wants to see you."

I remember thinking to myself, "But I don't want to go see Scott." I was scared of seeing death, of seeing "the unknown."

Boy, was Morrie Schwartz, Brandeis professor, ALS victim and hero of Mitch Albom's book **Tuesdays with Morrie**, correct in saying: "You have to know how to die to know how to live."

A friend said, "Barry, a dying man wants to talk to you. You must go."

Go I did, and, God, I got so much from the experience. Spending time with Scott and Hillary gave me so much better an appreciation of life and helped me truly understand why giving back is such a powerful and rewarding experience. I watched Hillary taking care of her dying husband, while telling me how lucky a person she was. She said, very matter-of-factly, how lucky she was to have married Scott…not just because of the time she treasured with him but also because of all the many, wonderful people who'd come into her life.

I've thought about that often. I think of how lucky I have been to meet so many wonderful people, too, and to have an opportunity to make a difference. Sometimes, it seems to me, we do not recognize an opportunity to take advantage of a situation that may change our lives…and that's when one of those wonderful people can step in, if we've allowed them into our lives. If I had not let Dennis Tetreault convince me to run the marathon, I would not have the job I have today. And I would not have traveled to Paris, London, Rome, Venice, Florence and Anguila. And I would not have met Matt, Meg, Skip, Jake and Sparky, Rat, and Scott and Hillary Carlson. Yes, I can hear them all now.

It was during this journey that I found myself sitting, at an Angel

Fund dinner, between Jake and Sparky Kennedy (who are family to me), and they were talking about how more and more cases of ALS have proven to somehow involve heredity. Looking into Sparky's eyes, I saw how scared she is. I felt like crying…I felt like I had to do something. It was then I knew I wanted to help in the fight to find a cure. There has to be an end to all this suffering.

This is why I believe the communication is complete for me: I know they can hear me, and I can hear them. Every Thursday night, I can still hear "Go, Liver Guy!" and I think of Scott and know he is out there, looking out for all his fellow runners, pushing us to strive to be the best that we can be.

I remember, too, during my first marathon…at around Mile 22…I did not have any feeling in either of my legs. I had come so far…and was not going to be able to crawl across the finish line. I honestly believe a special angel, Zelda, was cheering me on from above; God let her come down to massage my calf muscles. She could hear me then, and, when there is a problem and I need her, I can hear her.

To those who are not as lucky as I am, I feel an obligation to help promote the fight to find a cure. We must find the strength possessed by those people like Scott Carlson, Jimmy "The Squirrel" Kennedy and all the others who have succumbed to this terrible disease. They give us strength to fight the battle…if only we will listen to them.

I know I can hear them…and I pray that they hear me: We will make a difference.

By Paul DelVecchio

The Angel Fund views charitable donations not as money, but as gifts from God as we strive to find a cure for ALS. The Angel Fund's voice says, "With God Nothing is Impossible", the spirit and motto of our founder and the Angel Fund family, my wife (Ginny DelVecchio). Ginny truly had a never give up spirit, she was known to many as an "Angel of Inspiration", hence the name, Angel Fund. No one should ever feel alone in fighting the battle against ALS.

The Angel Fund brings awareness to the disease along with raising funds for research. With each fund-raising event and campaign, the fund contributes more and more money towards research which I feel is the means to the end of this disease. Over the years, I have known many patients, their families and friends, who emphasized that research to find a cure is their primary goal.

The Angel Fund can be heard on radio, seen on television, billboards etc. in attempting to accomplish its mission. The day the cure is found, is the day the Angel Fund closes. That day will be one of the most fulfilling days of my life.

Where do I begin? My mother, Ginny DelVecchio, is someone who was not easy to describe, nor was she predictable in any way. However, my purpose for this passage is to give you a chance to understand what I consider to be her strongest and most respectable quality, perhaps the most respectable any human being can possess.

Growing up with my mother was not easy for me; we had very different personalities and did not see things eye-to-eye many, many times. In fact, there were times that silence was the only solution to an issue. She and her Sicilian temper…me, with my lack of response to it; we were completely incompatible. Over the years our common stubbornness kept this stand-off well in place. However, my point of view changed over a most unlikely series of events, particularly concerning my work with my first mentor in my career field.

It all started when I was working as a civil servant for the State of Massachusetts. Since I was educated and licensed as a civil engineer, I found myself in my first full-time job as a field inspector, inspecting construction jobs. After my employers learned that I could touch type I was quickly moved to an administrative job. There I continue to change disciplines and started designing roadway projects. This eventually turned into more of a technology position as my lack of attention span pushed me into more high-tech, computer-related work with civil engineering and data collection. Eventually, I gravitated to the information technology world. Here I met and worked with my first mentor, a true visionary. More appropriately, I stumbled upon this mentor.

I first would like to say that I consider myself privileged to have worked with and know this person. He was a special advisor to the chief engineer working with the field inspectors. He knew the struggles and downfalls of this group of workers, who were often ignored and under-rated, and he saw through the politics to refocus much needed resources. He believed that a change was needed to aid workers with better tools to help them perform their jobs more effectively and efficiently.

My role in this vision was to design, construct and implement the technology tools to make this vision a reality. The opportunity and experience has not and is not expected to be equaled again. By working with this man and the field workers, I learned to communicate and work with a wide variety of people and their problems.

More importantly, this man taught and demonstrated the characteristics of a true public servant. He was a former Marine who fought in World War II. He was all about honesty, righteousness and working to serve the public directly or indirectly through the work we were doing – in much the same way as he had served his country during his military career. I subscribed this philosophy whole-heartedly; I learned to understand the role and importance of civil servitude. Today, as I write this, I have not forgotten the valuable lessons learned and continue my work as a public servant.

It was this philosophy that connected my mother and me. I never fully realized that she had adopted a similar philosophy to the one I acquired through my professional mentor. During the time her mother contracted ALS, she started the Massachusetts Chapter for ALS, and spurred the other New England states to do the same, often spending hundreds of hours on the phone talking to people. More than just instrumentally helping to create these much-needed support organizations, she spent countless hours talking to and educating afflicted patients and their families about ALS, and about what resources were available to them. Most of the time she would communicate with these people just to let them know that they were not alone, and to never give up hope.

After she contracted ALS her motherly instincts kicked into high gear. She told me that she would do everything she could to ensure that my brother and I would not be another victim of ALS.

And it was so ironic that this most dedicated supporter of ridding the world of ALS now found herself as an ALS patient in need of support; amazingly, she continued her work at the front of the battle. She believed that the most effective way to keep her promise to me was to find a cure through research, hence the creation of the Angel Fund. She believed that by bringing about greater awareness of ALS, and by focusing efforts on research, that she could better help the ALS community eradicate this insidious disease.

During her long four years fighting for her life with this disease, her motivation to promote, support and try new things caused her unspeakable pain and suffering – to an extent I had never seen before and pray never to see again. Her aim became to destroy ALS, not just for my brother and I, but for everyone. She promoted awareness through public appearances and interviews. She tried countless drugs, inventive medical techniques, and was involved in experimental medical trials. All of these were extremely hard on her, both physically and mentally because of her debilitating physical condition and her first-hand knowledge of the disease.

At the very end she died with respect, thinking of others even in her final hours, in the true spirit of considering herself last and thinking about what was best for those closest to her.

Just after her last living moment I remember thinking: "There goes a true public servant, my other mentor, my mother."

On one final note, I would like to take this opportunity to thank each and every nurse, caregiver, doctor, friend and family member who aided our family in taking care of my mother when she was ill with ALS. And to all of the people that have supported the Angel Fund or any ALS support organization, bless your heart.

By Kim DiRocco

My story begins in the fall of 1999. My name is Kim DiRocco and I am a respiratory therapist. I live in Tewksbury, with my husband, Todd, and our two boys, Zak and Alex. How I got involved with the Angel Fund has been one, incredible journey.

As I said, it began in 1999…when my husband was visiting a friend of ours from high school, a friend named Willie. He'd been recently diagnosed with ALS. Although we had not been in much contact with Willie since high school, it was devastating to learn that he was diagnosed with this horrific disease. He was only 33 years old at the time.

Because of my profession I knew more about this disease, and its terrible path ahead, than any of our friends. After a few visits with Willie, my husband would come home and update me on his condition. Those visits would usually take place on Tuesdays; we began calling his visits "Tuesdays with Willie," just like the title of the book, **Tuesdays with Morrie** (which has become one of my favorite books).

As a respiratory therapist and as the type of person who can't resist being a friend of someone in need, I mentioned to Todd that he should, on his next visit, mention to our friend Willie that if he ever needed me to answer any questions about his disease, or to assist in his care, that I would go to his home.

Within two weeks I found myself at his home, offering my professional care to this friend in need. This developed into a strong friendship with not only Willie, but also his parents, Kay and Bill. To this day we talk weekly. Having two sons of my own, I could only imagine the pain that they, too, were suffering.

I changed my shift daytime on Thursdays at the hospital so I could care for Willie during the day and go to work for the evening shift. Thursdays became my day with Willie.

I began caring for him on a weekly basis. I knew this was not a lifetime commitment. I had tremendous support from my family: my husband, my boys, mother and father-in-law, my sister-in-law, and all my friends.

Thus it was that I was with Willie, along with his family, on the night he died…April 13, 2000. It was one of the nights I happened to sleep at his house because I did not feel comfortable leaving him.

During the months leading to Willie's death, I researched and learned more about ALS. But most of what I learned about was becoming comfortable with talking to someone who is dying. And we talked a lot about that. No textbook could teach me how to really listen to someone. That developed through friendship and trust and these elements, I think, are what made our relationship unique.

I can recall one night caring for Willie and feeding him Junior Mints as we watched a movie. I thought of this as a simple task but suddenly came to realize that it was a much bigger thing to me as he turned to me and said, in his slurred speech: "You're such a good friend."

Understanding Willie was becoming more and more difficult for most; although I found the more time spent with him the easier it was to understand him. Sort of like a helpless child, who only a mother knows what he or she wants. This is how I became dedicated to his care. Like a mother, caring for a child.

After thinking long and hard about what small gift I could give him for Christmas, I decided to make him a blanket. I thought about how difficult it is for some people to visit, for fear they would not understand him. I also thought about how difficult it is for some people to have a conversation with someone who is dying. So, I had his family gather many pictures and then transferred them on to this blanket. Then, when people visited they could look at and talk about the pictures…when they did not know what else to say. If they could only hear me seems so appropriate, as a heart-breaking communication concern, in such situations.

Now, his mother keeps this blanket on her bed.

I remember sleeping at the hospital when Willie would be admitted because we were afraid that even the nurses were not familiar with caring for ALS patients, such as knowing how to move them, understand them, or just know their most comfortable positions. Many are not. This is one of the reasons why I hope to continue my work on trying to educate healthcare providers in hospitals and those who provide care at home, for ALS patients, about how to care for these particularly fragile human beings. This is a work in progress, but I hope to be in contact with the right people that will help me to put such a program together and make it available.

Awareness about this disease is so important. This is why, after Willie died, I knew I wanted to continue to try and make a difference. I also think it is so important that people should do something for others in their lives – whatever it is that makes you feel you helped someone other than yourself. There's a rewarding sense of feeling appreciation that others have for us, and a great feeling that comes from that "sense of giving," and that sense of "being a good person" when we do something like this. It's really not so difficult.

I chose to join the fight against ALS because I found such a huge lack of knowledge about this disease. People are just not fully aware what this disease is really all about; mostly, I think, because death occurs too quickly once diagnosed. I really feel the need to do my part, in every way I can, to help bring this awareness forward.

In caring for Willie I felt as though I was simply able to offer something that came so easy to me…but, clearly, meant so much to him physically and emotionally. Although it was at times strenuous, taxing my own personal life, I would do it again tomorrow if I am needed. I could never explain the gratitude and sense of appreciation that I felt coming my way because I cared for someone so debilitated by this horrific disease. Just knowing I could offer comfort and make a difference in this unfortunate journey taken by someone else has, in a very real sense, changed my life. I understand now that every little bit that people can do, in offering something of themselves, can make a tremendous difference to someone else.

In a world where material things matter so very much, I know I made a difference in someone's life by simply providing dedication, care and friendship. Money cannot buy this. I was greatly appreciated by someone in need: What greater payment or gift could there be?

One day, in May of 2000, just one month after Willie died, I was reading a newspaper and came across an advertisement for the Angel Fund. I had never heard of the Angel Fund before and, as I read, I learned about the organization and its goals. I called and spoke to the fund's executive director, Paul DelVecchio, my mind racing the entire time. Thoughts were triggered left and right as I realized immediately: "Here's my way of becoming involved and finding ways to develop awareness of this disease." I did, however, wonder: "How am I going to tell my family what I am about to do?"

After learning more about the Angel Fund, I decided to hold a golf tournament, devoted to the cause of promoting awareness of ALS. Sure enough, my family and friends were not surprised.

I do remember Paul saying: "It's not every day I receive a phone call from someone saying they want to hold a golf tournament and donate all the money to the Angel Fund." At the time, the fund was just a few years old; but each year it has grown, adding more and more events.

I have found the Angel Fund to be a truly unique organization. I very much appreciate that is managed by a small group of individuals, who do not profit from any of the contributions. All the money raised goes toward research and awareness.

I am grateful I have found the Angel Fund, to continue my efforts and to communicate with patients and families on its website.

I have met so many great individuals through the Angel Fund. Everyone is like family.

I have found my "sense of giving" and I continue to use it through the Angel Fund.

I now dedicate my time to the Angel Fund, supporting its efforts to keep the memories alive of those we have lost, and to support the many others who are still suffering from this horrible disease.

This year, along with the help of family and friends, we will hold our Fourth Annual Angel Fund/Lou Gehrig's Disease Awareness Golf Tournament.

Each year I come into contact with more and more individuals and families afflicted by this disease, as well as those we have lost, and I add their names to the golf tournament packet. I can only hope that some day, soon, this list will get smaller rather than bigger.

People still ask me, "Kim, why did you do what you did for Willie? Why are you continuing to work for the Angel Fund?"

And I say, "It's simple. Because I can!" Working hard at something is easy when you truly believe in what you are doing.

I once read a quote…but now I truly understand it:

Friends are Angels who lift our wings

when we have difficulty

remembering how to fly.

By Sal Falzone

I wrestled with writing about what ALS and the Angel Fund mean to me. I dodged this project for many months – not because I wanted to avoid considering what has driven me to be involved with the ALS cause for so many years, but merely because my story is so simple.

You see, I have not gone through the ultimate tests of faith, hope and love that are required of those who have ALS or those who are close to somebody with this death sentence. I have been very lucky, so far, spared of the day-to-day challenges these folks need to face. I have no idea how I would get through such a challenge, but I would say that it would change nearly every facet of my life.

Many victims of this horrible disease manage to find within themselves the strength to view everything in the most positive ways. This should be the ultimate goal of all of us, to be sure, although few of us accomplish it. We all know stories about people who, seemingly against all odds, prevail. Why? I think there is something amazing that can happen when people face their toughest tests. Some find that they have the goods. They have within them all the answers about survival, even in their dying. They set extraordinary examples for all of us to ponder and try to learn from.

I will give a short answer to the following question: Why, when there are so many other ways to spend your free time, do you continue to put your energy and skills into the ALS cause?

I believe it is healthy for me to try to help others; I believe I bring objectivity to the cause, being a CPA and one of very few individuals involved in the Angel Fund community who has not been struck by ALS in my household. Tragically, the demand far exceeds the supply.

It certainly would be a lot more entertaining for me to be on the board of a non-profit organization in, say, the Arts. Of course, this is not to take anything away at all from those on such boards; many such board members serve on multiple boards and promote great and worthy achievements. But for me, it is different. God knows, I find it challenging enough to earn my living, help keep my firm growing, and help raise my family the best I know how. But I also feel compelled to give back to the community in some way – and this cause is where I have chosen to make a contribution and where I feel I can make the most difference. The cause is certainly an important one and as long as the efforts and integrity remain to move the cause forward, I feel good about continuing my efforts.

Ginny DelVecchio was a beautiful person, as anybody who knew her will attest. This inner beauty did not tarnish with the onset or progression of the disease. There are many people, like Ginny, who have their acts together; there are many, many more who hope they do, and never know until they are tested. My hope is that more of us will discover we are made of such stuff that we could hold up under such a test, but that we will never have to go through such a thing, particularly so terrible a disease as ALS.

By Anne T. Fucillo

I first met Ginny when our sons were playing baseball for Merrimack College. We spent many games together and even traveled to Florida together with our families during spring training.

At the games, while she cheered on the boys, she would be stuffing envelopes with letters that she was mailing out to people who had lost loved ones to ALS. She had started a support group because she had lost a mother and brother to the disease. She knew what these people were going through.

I knew very little about ALS before I met Ginny. But like the many others she touched, I learned a lot about the disease and about living from her.

I believe that the Angel Fund was a dream of hers that came to life. Her hope stirred the people who came into contact with her. And her drive for a cure reached many more people, through various fund-raisers and news stories. Even when she was sick she seemed to radiate a peace that put those around her at ease. She was never thinking about herself but, instead, she focused on the future and how she could help find a cure for this terrible disease.

Ginny was a warm, loving person, with a wonderful laugh – she truly enjoyed life. I am so fortunate to have been her friend and I treasure the memories I had with her.

She had such a strong faith in God; I believe that He needed an angel on earth to help raise awareness, to comfort others who have suffered from ALS, and to work to find a cure.

Ginny was that angel.

By Roberta "Bobbi" Gibb

(Editor's note: Bobbi Gibb, a local, young Winchester, Massachusetts resident, stunned the running world when she became the first woman ever to run and complete the 26.2-mile Boston Marathon on April 19, 1966. Prevailing beliefs, until Bobbi proved them all totally wrong, were that women were not physiologically capable of running anything longer than 3.1 miles. Though women were not "officially" allowed to enter the Boston Marathon until 1972, today, the Boston Marathon recognizes Bobbi Gibb not only as the first woman to run Boston but as the official women's winner of the 1966, 1967 and 1968 Boston Marathons.)

Two men walked up my driveway. One was wearing a colorful windbreaker and a big smile; the other was dressed in a suit and appeared to be more reserved. Little did I know that I was about to meet two Angels.

I'd always thought that Angels were ethereal beings – you know, beings with long, white wings, who dwell in the clouds above the fray. But here they were – solid guys. Paul DelVecchio, executive director of the Angel Fund, was the man who reached out his hand to give me a warm handshake. He introduced Sinclair, a lawyer and philanthropist, who looked at me, with those intense, crystal blue eyes of his.

It was April 2001. I had come home, to run the Boston Marathon in celebration of the 35th anniversary of my first run in 1966…

Before my run in 1966 it had been thought that women were not able to complete the marathon distance; furthermore, they were not allowed to try. So my run, in 1966, was a challenge to authority – the race authorities who accepted only male applications to compete in the race and all those self-appointed "authorities" who set limits on what females can be expected to do. I'd hoped my race would change the way men thought about women, and, equally important, I'd hoped it would change the way women thought about themselves.

On Patriots Day, April 19, 1966, I had hid in the bushes near the start of the marathon in Hopkinton, fearful race officials would actually have me arrested for breaking the rule of "no women allowed." And when the starting gun was fired I jumped into the pack, and ran all the way to Boston, in a time of 3 hours and 20 minutes, finishing ahead of two-thirds of the men, a feat which made headlines around the world.

My finish was, literally, front-page headlines in Boston the next day. It excites me, still, to think about how beautifully my effort fit in, in the world-wide effort that was afoot to galvanize women. For, it was just two months later that the National Organization of Women (NOW) was founded and the women's movement began in earnest. It was gratifying to see my run discussed frequently in the following terms: If women could do something like this, something previously thought impossible, what else could women do?! Maybe they could be…doctors, lawyers, senators, representatives, board members, CEOs, astronauts! The next year I ran the Boston Marathon again, and the next year, continuing the battle and making my personal statement on this subject. More and more women began to run. And, for many women, running was the first step towards developing a greater sense of personal self-confidence and autonomy.

I had come to running from a feeling there was something missing in the lifestyle the Sixties had laid out for me. I found in running a healing, meditative spirit, which I wanted to share with others to open up the possibility of running as a way of healing ourselves and our culture. Running, I had found, helps bind mind, body and soul back into a natural unity.

The Boston Marathon has become my "second family" over the years, and I've felt blessed by the multitude of friendships I've found through running…

Now, 35 years later, I was running again, hoping to raise money to fight ALS, a tragic, paralytic disease that was now affecting one of my dearest friends, Buck.

I sensed already that I was about to find another family — a family of Angels.

The association began with Ed Rice, who told me about the Angel Fund. Ed was one of the founders of the Angel Fund and a friend of Ginny DelVecchio, the original Angel and inspiration for the fund. He had joined her and her husband, Paul, to focus attention on Ginny's heroic struggle against ALS. As the editor of the Winchester Town Crier, he'd documented Ginny's story, trying to support her in the effort to educate the public about ALS and the need to support ALS research. During the time of Ginny's battle with ALS Ed had published article after article about her, her indomitable spirit, her love, the love of the people around her, her faith in God. It was around this same time that people in the greater Boston area were growing excited about the approach of the 100th anniversary of the Boston Marathon.

Knowing that I had grown up in Winchester, Ed had called me, to do an interview about my history with the run. Ultimately, he produced an excellently-written article.

We had stayed in touch. Now, in 2001, Ed was looking for a way to run Boston again, in order to continue to call public attention to the fight against ALS, and I invited him to join me for the run. I had wanted to do something to help Massachusetts General Hospital, to show my appreciation because the hospital had been so extraordinarily good to one of my closest friends, Charles, whom I'd taken care of in my home as he struggled with cancer and died in 1993.

When I mentioned to Ed that one of my best friends, Buck, had contracted ALS, he responded by telling me Ginny's story. I was moved and decided to join the Angel Fund and the group of runners running the marathon on behalf of the fund. It was then that I met Scott and Hillary Carlson. I was touched by the love I felt between these two remarkable people: Hillary, Scott's athletic soul mate and new bride, and Scott, once an outstanding athlete, now strickened with the dread disease. Courageously they faced ALS together.

Soon more of the Angels appeared: Lisa Courtenay, the Angel Fund administrator who works tirelessly on behalf of the fund in the law offices of Eugene Nigro; Eugene, a director of the fund who donates office space, staff and other resources for the fund; Richard Kennedy, president of the Angel Fund, whose and father and brother died of ALS; and then, of course, Dr. Robert Brown, whose research laboratory is funded by the Angel Fund, and who is, quite simply, an extraordinary man.

These Angels are not ethereal beings who live in the clouds free of human struggle. All of these remarkable people have had their own battles to fight, their own slings and arrows and wounds, and have overcome sometimes overwhelming difficulties with courage and integrity. Yet, these people, these Angels, all take the time to care about and to work hard and give of themselves to help others and this is what makes them, each one of them, a hero. As I have become closer to them I have come to love and admire them for their immense humanity, humility, dedication and compassion.

I think of the Bible passage from Corinthians: "Though ye speak with the tongue of men and angels and have not charity, thee become as sounding brass or a tinkling cymbal… "And though ye have the gift of prophesy and understand all mysteries, and all knowledge, and though ye have all faith, so that ye can move mountains and have not charity, ye are nothing." These human Angels have this quality of compassion and charity and this is the foundation of each of their lives and the foundation of the Angel Fund.

After training all winter in California, of course, I had come down with the flu in March. I was taking massive doses of vitamin C as

I appeared on television shows and was interviewed for magazine and newspaper articles to reminisce about that first run back in 1966. But I made a point, each and every time, to tell about the Angel Fund and why I was running the Boston Marathon again. The day finally came. Ed Rice, my running companion in this adventure, and I took the bus with the elite runners from the Copley Plaza in Boston to the start in Hopkinton, accompanied by a cavalcade of motorcycle police with blue lights flashing and sirens screaming. Sadly much of this pageantry was lost on me: I was coughing and hacking, with a case of bronchitis, and felt utterly drained of energy.

We arrived in Hopkinton long before the start with thousands of other runners, all of whom milled around stretching, talking, drinking fluids. Excitement hung in the air between the bare trees, the old New England houses, and the groups of spectators, all under the stark, brilliant sky.

I was delighted to see my friend, Dr. Harvey Weinstein. He devotes himself to directing the children's oncology ward at Massachusetts General Hospital and still takes the time to train for and run the Boston Marathon to raise money to fight children's cancer. The stalwart members of the Boston Police Running Club were also here. These policemen and policewomen, who serve in one of the toughest jobs one can imagine, and then, on their time off, what do they do? Train to run the Boston Marathon to fight cancer, ALS and other devastating diseases. Harvey watched in amusement as I cut the side panels off my running shoes, so my little toes would have space. He still teases me about it.

Ed and I placed ourselves way back in the pack of runners. It was a warm sunny day. Even so I was wearing leotards because I knew I would be going slowly. I just didn't know, yet, how slowly. Ed was daringly dressed in short shorts and a skimpy singlet. The starting gun was fired. The front runners broke and gradually the wave of motion spread backwards until we too began to move. Already I could feel that this was another triumph of organization for race director Dave McGillivray, executive director Guy Morse, and the entire BAA! Like a well-orchestrated dance the choreographed start proceeded in perfect harmony. I caught a glimpse of Hillary and the other runners who were running for Scott and the Angel Fund.

We ran on and on through the familiar markers along the familiar roads hardly looking at our surroundings, concentrating on the keeping the rhythm of our own running, conscious only of the runners around us, the sounds of our footsteps, the pavement, the way we all feel together running like this. Just as in life we are surrounded by people but we still have to do the running ourselves. We are doing what we love, which makes us happy, and we're doing it for others, which makes us even happier.

At the halfway mark in Wellesley I felt very sick. Feverish and dizzy I wanted to stop but I couldn't: I was determined to keep running for the Angel Fund. I couldn't let these people down. They worked every day, every year, and they were expecting me to run to the finish and to be at the race-end gathering at the Park Plaza. It was there that I would have the honor of meeting Dr. Brown, one of the best-known researchers and physicians dealing directly with ALS in the world. My friend, Buck, was waiting for me there. And it was there where I would see the Angels again: Sinclair, Paul, Lisa, Tom, Eugene, Scott, Hillary…plus more I'd yet to meet.

My body felt like lead. I felt faint. Every few minutes I'd say to Ed, "If I pass out, just drag me over to the side." Or some other similarly "encouraging" statement. I felt so heavy. I was so tired that there was, it seemed to me, a pause between when my brain give the signal and when my legs actually moved. I thought of my grandfather, who was a tough old Scot, like Jock Semple, the grandfather of BAA for many years. And I thought of Ed running with me now.

Ed is a true gentlemen and I will always be grateful to him for this. My pace was so slow that Ed could have easily walked beside me, but he did not. He kept up the appearance of running, almost in place at times. And I reworded that old joke about the definition of a gentleman as it was told to me: The definition of a gentleman is one who can walk but keeps on running so the lady doesn't look completely ridiculous. Ed, bless his soul, jogged beside me as I dragged my sick body along, wheezing and coughing, teetering on the verge of unconsciousness and collapse. I'd feel a blackness pass over me and I struggled to keep from passing out. He jogged beside me even though it would have been easier for him to walk.

We began to run from tree to tree, meaning we'd sight a tree down the road and focus just on running to that tree. Never mind about the twelve more miles on the other side of the tree! As I staggered by, we were both smiling and waving to people, people who were calling out: "Yea, ALS! Yea, Angel Fund!"; "My Dad had ALS"; "My mother died of ALS"; "My brother's got ALS"; "My best friend had ALS." So many peoples' lives have been touched by this tragic and inexplicable disease, which cuts a huge swathe in the lives of everyone involved, as the dread disease progresses for three to five years, leaving the survivors almost bankrupted by the expense of it, exhausted, often with post traumatic stress syndrome, as if they'd been through a war. These Angels have been through their own wars, all of them. The least I could do, I tried to reason with myself, was to finish this marathon for them.

On I ran, barely able to stand up, painfully pulling each leg, by shear force of will, in front of the next until, finally, we were over Heart-break Hill. I'd made it up and over the top and looked over at Ed, who was turning blue with chills. A crisp, cold headwind had sprung up and was blowing easterly from the ocean. Ed was freezing in his singlet and shorts. "Go on ahead," I shouted.

"Are you sure?" he shouted back.

"Yes, you're freezing I'll be fine. I'll get on the medical truck and see you at the finish," I said. So Ed sprinted off, glad to be released, but bothered by feelings of guilt. I staggered to the medical bus and collapsed: my lungs felt full of sawdust; my stomach felt like a rotten fish; my legs cramped up; and I doubled over the chair, pressing the back of the chair into my stomach to ease the pain. I stayed like that hanging over the chair, as the bus lurched forward and went very fast, swaying crazily from side to side, accelerating, then screeching on the brakes at every stop light, as if possessed. We headed west, back up the course, all the way back to Wellesley, the halfway mark. Then we turned around and began picking up stragglers and volunteers on the way back. After about 40 minutes of sway-ing and jerking, and nauseated by the smell of diesel fuel, I discovered the cramp in my gut had loosened and I could breathe again. In fact, I started feeling pretty good again, after the rest and after drinking some water.

As we approached the very place where I had boarded the bus some 45 minutes ago, I began to feel the challenge stirring in me. Again. I just couldn't NOT finish this race. Look at what the Angels did! The least I could do was to finish this race for them!

"Stop the bus!" I shouted. The bus jerked to a stop and I leaped out.

Sizing up my condition and something more, a young woman jumped off with me. "I know who you are," she said to me, "…what your place is in the history of this race. It would be an honor for me to run with you." She was a volunteer dressed, not in running clothes, but in jeans. Even so she ran with me. My pace was better now and there were about five more miles, I figured, to the finish.

We ran along stride for stride, talking a bit. Her name, she said, was Rebecca Wolfe. She was a grad student at Harvard, just finishing up. And she was training to run a marathon in Tennessee.

Around us, the last remnants of the race were collapsing. A sea of empty paper cups, which carpeted the road in front of each disassembled water station, was being swept away by people with brooms. The water tables had been folded up and there was no water to be had. Ropes that had held the crowd back were being coiled up, and traffic was moving on the street again. I'd never seen the back end of the race before.

We descended past the graveyard and ran parallel to the trolley line on Commonwealth Avenue, then through familiar Coolidge Corner and on into Boston. We were dodging the cars on the streets, running up on the sidewalks, darting in and out of crowds of young people who were headed for the pubs. "Excuse us…Excuse us…Sorry…Oops!" We tried to be polite, especially when people made an effort to let us pass without breaking our momentum. "Thanks." Up and down the curbs we danced. The huge red Citgo sign loomed over us, as it always does, and seemed to stay there hanging for an interminable length of time as we slogged down Beacon and, ultimately, through Kenmore Square.

Strangely, this was the best I'd felt the entire race. My pace had picked up and I felt in amazingly good spirits. I thought about the Angel Fund party going on, about Buck and Paul, Lisa and Sinclair and Dr. Brown, who I still looking forward to meeting. I thought about Sinclair, who loved to help people, despite his own struggles, and his fund, well-named the Good Samaritans, dedicated to doing good for others. The Samaritan was the one who had stopped to help, when others passed by, and I felt touched. Later, Sinclair told me that the subject of "Where is Bobbi?" kept coming up, and they'd correctly surmised that I might be still out on the course.

Finally, Rebecca and I made the turn right on to Hereford Street, into a canyon of brick buildings, and then left on to Boylston, into the openness, and the relief. The finish was in view and the line from the Bible came to me, "And behold, there are the last which shall be first and there are the first which shall be last." I thought about my first run 35 years ago that had opened people's minds and hearts to running and to the world of possibilities. I had found something through my running that I hoped others would find and I'd helped change the way people thought about women. I remembered how I was then, young, at the beginning of my life, not knowing what the future would bring. I thought of my own innocence. How unprepared I was for my reception as the crowds screamed wildly, the press crowded around me, and the Governor of Massachusetts himself came up to me at the finish line to shake my hand. Now, the crowds are gone, the grandstands are being folded up, the street is empty, except for the litter on the grey pavement.

Tears rolled down my face as I felt the effects of achievement, resulting from a tremendous effort: I've done it again. These tears seemed appropriate as I contemplated the poignancy of the passage of time for me, for all of us. They were tears of love for this running life I love so much, for all the people in it I love. Two huge, orange, street sweepers, as if on cue, noisily started up and escorted us majestically down the street to the finish. The humor and the irony of it prompted me to double over with laughter, and Rebecca laughed too. As we passed the official timing clock for the marathon, I glanced up and saw that it was dead, desolate, dark. It was stopped at 6 o'clock, the deadline set as the time limit for all competitors to complete the race.

We made our way to the Copley Plaza Hotel, where the awards ceremony was being held. We opened the doors and walked into the lobby, but right then I collapsed, unable to breathe. A nurse grabbed me and tried to get me to put my head down. "No, no," I said, "I need to go outside again." I wrenched myself free, ran outside and began running up and down the sidewalk. When I was running I could breathe; when I stopped running I couldn't breathe. Rebecca ran out after me, and I put my hand on her shoulder as we jogged up and down the street to avoid running into people. Finally, I was able to breathe. Ultimately I slowed down to a walk and, after 20 minutes, went in for the end of the awards ceremony.

Author, stellar runner and coach, and friend, Tom Derderian came over to me and we watched together. Then, just as I was about to leave, I saw Ed sitting on the carpeted stair, still in his running clothes, with one of those shiny metallic space blankets volunteers give entrants at the finish line pulled around him to keep him warm. "Ed!" I cried. "How are you? What was your time?"

He told me he'd broken the six-hour barrier and gotten a finishing medal, and then apologized for leaving me.

"No, no it was fine. I wanted you to finish. How did you know I'd be so stupid as to jump off the bus and run the whole thing?" I protested. "No it's not your fault. If it hadn't been for you I wouldn't have run. I wouldn't have met the Angels... I suppose their gathering is over?"

"Long over," he said. We used my accommodations at the hotel to clean up, and then we sat down to a pasta dinner together.

In all, the runners raised some $110,000 in contributions for Dr. Brown's lab. This was my introduction to the Angel Fund.

Several months later, Sinclair was kind enough to take me to visit Dr. Brown and his lab, and I began to understand something about what the disease of ALS is all about. Dr. Brown impressed me tremendously, with his intelligence and compassion and dedication. ALS is, truly, a mystery and it intrigued me then and intrigues me still. I began to study my biochemistry again. I'd been a pre-med major in college but had gone on to become a lawyer, and to practice law, for many years; but biology remains one of my loves. The more I read, the more mystified I became. I sent my letters of ideas, insights, questions, and puzzlements to Dr. Brown who, despite the huge demands on his time, was kind enough to respond and to encourage me. We met again that fall and again the next spring. Each time my understanding of ALS was increasing and I documented the progress he was making in the lab, and writing about it in lay person's English for Angel Fund publications, for the benefit of their funding sources.

The next year, 2002, I didn't run, but worked with Lisa to write the grant which was sent out to over 100 foundations and corporations. Sinclair's questions and his compassion and generosity have, clearly, been major factors in the Angel Fund's success.

Knowing these people, who devote their time and energy to raising money for research about and treatment of ALS, and to helping those afflicted, makes me feel humble and moved.

Since then Scott Carlson has passed away; yet I treasure my friendship with his wife, Hillary.

Last summer, in 2003, I spent considerable time with my friend Buck, who was dying of ALS. My roles were caring for him and giving breaks to his wonderful wife, Caroline, who was struggling herself with breast cancer. Of course, there were excellent nurses and caretakers for him, too.

Buck loved to laugh. Even when nearly his entire body was paralyzed, except for his arms and hands, and his head, he regaled us with spicy jokes and stories. On one of our expeditions, he wanted to see "Johnny English," a comedy with Rowan Atkinson, who is usually known as "Mr. Bean." I drove Buck's van, which had been fitted out to accommodate his wheel chair. We had a quick lunch, drove to the theater and parked. We opened the automated door, with its automated ramp, which we laughingly compared to the "Star Wars" space shuttle, and wheeled the chair down the ramp and into the movie theater. It gave me a glimpse into the challenges that the handicapped have to meet on a daily basis. Once in the theater, we ate popcorn and howled with laughter at the antics of this comic British actor. After the film we went out to dinner and, again, the logistics of simply getting in and out of a vehicle, which we take for granted, were formidable. Then we went home, which involved again helping Buck out of the van and into the house. From there, Buck required a difficult bathing and toiletry regime, and the use of a motorized pulley system and harness, for getting him in and out of the wheelchair and into bed. The shear physical effort of all this on a daily basis was incredible, and yet I could see he was keeping his mind, his personality intact. He so courageous in the face of all this.

I thought of Ginny DelVecchio and what she went through, and what her husband Paul, and family and friends went through with her, in this heart-breaking disease. Thinking about what every person with ALS suffers, and what those who love them and care for them suffer, makes me marvel at the shear strength and courage this disease requires.

On Sunday we went to church in Portsmouth, New Hampshire, Buck's favorite church. We attended the Unitarian Church service, held in this spacious, old stone building, with open ceiling and beams. I watched Buck's face. I turned away because I didn't want him to see I was crying. But tears were streaming down his face, too. I thought back over the 32 years we had known and loved each other, the projects we had worked on: the film on the environment and alternative energy we had made with Amory Lovins; the conservation work we'd done; and just the many hours in friendship we'd spent together. Somehow I had never thought of it ever ending...Not so soon ...Not like this.

Buck's best friend Hawkins, and Hawk's lovely wife, Lorrie, and their three beautiful children, Ashley, Juliet and Jenna, were there. After church we ate at a French restaurant with Buck's daughter, Sophie. We missed Winslow, Buck's son (who was named after Winslow Homer, Buck's favorite artist), and Caroline, who were away at a soccer game.

Somehow the normal, small things of life, the things you hardly notice when you're doing them — the way the sun floods through the window just so, the way someone you love smiles or looks sad, or suddenly takes your hand and holds it, pressing it hard against him — the small things turn out to be the most important, most precious things of all. Especially when time is running out and each week, each day, each moment seems filled with a poignant light, only temporarily keeping grief at bay.

And then finally when it comes, it is still unexpected. So soon? He seemed so well only yesterday, so full of life. Surely he had another six months, another year. What made him let go so fast? I called only yesterday and he was in the midst of a party, with all his friends, celebrating an anniversary for Cambridge Alternative Energy Company (CAPCO), a business he started some 25 years ago, now thriving. And the next day he's dead? How could it be possible? We had so much more yet to do. We were going to write some articles on the environment. We were going to see another spring, maybe spend the winter in St. John's. Death is so final.

Buck said he never thought much about what happens afterwards. It's over and that's the tragedy of it: Life was it.

By Ann Hadley

I have been involved with the Angel Fund for the past three years. My role in the Angel Fund Family (and, yes, it IS a family!) is that of a marketing/public relations consultant, hired to bring awareness about ALS research and to help raise funds.

Over the course of these three years I have met some amazing people. Their dedication to the fund and their perseverance in finding a cure are second to none. They are genuinely affected and concerned when another patient is diagnosed; they bring these patients and their loved ones into the Angel Fund family, letting them know they are not alone in this battle and, more importantly, letting them know that they, too, have fought this battle.

I see Rich Kennedy, Paul DelVecchio, Jan Nigro and Eugene Nigro working hard to raise money for research to win the battle and find a cure. They work on behalf of all families, like themselves, who have been affected by ALS, hoping that another member of their own family will not be the next victim of this horrendous disease.

Before working with the Angel Fund, I knew of the disease, but I never really knew the faces of ALS. Nor did I know about the short life expectancy or that, at the end of the disease, the mind is alert while the body has lost all muscle control.

I am honored to work alongside many of the people involved in the Angel Fund – those who conduct fund-raisers, those who have been personally affected by ALS. And those who have ALS. I will continue to work on their behalf because I have seen the horrible disease and the effects of the disease, not only on the patient, but also on their families. I am in awe of their courage.

The Angel Fund is founded on hope…the hope that a cure will be found.

Time is of the essence…for the ALS patient time is not on his or her side. Yet.

As an added bonus, I have gained many new friends – the many wonderful people who work day to day to raise funds to find the cure.

By Jillian Hensley

*(Editor's note: This story by Boston Globe reporter Jillian Hensley, first ap-
peared on the pages of the Globe and was subsequently printed in the Fall
2000 issue of the Angel Fund newsletter Angel Advocate. We are grateful
to the Boston Globe for the opportunity to reprint this story about the late
Scott Carlson. It is a fitting testimonial to his courage and that of his wife,
Hillary)*

"When the doctor says, 'Well, you have to think of death as a possibility,' all of a sudden everything comes crashing down, and you have to pull
yourself up. You make a decision right then: Am I going to stay down there,
or am I going to live my life. I choose to live my life."

-from Scott Carlson's diary

*(Editor's note: In May, 1998, Scott Carlson, after numerous tests, had to
confront the possibility that he had ALS. When Dr. Cudkwicz at MGH
took over his case in September of that year, ALS was almost a certainty.
The official diagnosis came in February, 1999…the month in which he and
Hillary married and bought their house.)*

T ucked away on a dead-end street in Warwick, Rhode Island,
within sound and scent of the sea, is a brown Cape-style house, the home
of Scott and Hillary Carlson, and their red setter, Diego.

As the doorbell rings, Diego, self-appointed official greeter,
bounds to the glass storm door, closely followed by a smiling Hillary. Diego
sniffs and wags and grins, making sure that the visitors are no threat to his
household. Hillary calls, "Scott, we have guests."

Emerging from his den, Scott greets us warmly, using his left
hand. He looks much younger than his 37 years.

We move into the living room, where Scott lies back in a well-pad-
ded recliner. A handmade guitar and a tall, narrow cabinet full of guitar-
greats memorabilia testify to his passion for music. On walls and furniture,
photos, of happy times shared with Hillary and with friends and family,
offer glimpses into his life. Many of the pictures reflect the enthusiasm he
and Hillary share for athletics. They met in August 1997, when Hillary was
life-guarding a triathlon in which Scott was competing. It was to be his
last. He had detected weakness in his right arm a few months before. On
February 23, 1999, they eloped.

Hillary's love for her husband and her pride in all he continues to achieve are palpable. In the months before their marriage, when they were going to the doctor every week for a new test, they had a long time to think about what it all meant.

"There was never any question in my mind and heart that he was the person I wanted to be with. Nothing would come between him and my love. What many people don't realize is that we both have the disease. It affects both of us profoundly, but we work really well together and ALS has made us better people. Of course, I never thought I'd be having this kind of experience at this time of my life – giving IVs, for instance – but I don't want to be anywhere else."

She and Scott agree that the self-discipline and ability to focus that he developed through athletic training and playing guitar have been major factors in helping him to cope with the progression of the disease. "He's a perfectionist," she says. "He won't settle for anything less. That plays a major role in his life."

"Before, I was so focused on physical capabilities and trying to improve them that when all those things stopped, I was faced with a huge lifestyle change," Scott explains. "So, how do you adapt to that? 'Well,' I said, 'there are all these things I never did before so I might as well enjoy them while I can.'"

Reading now features prominently on his agenda, and is catching up on books he never had an opportunity to explore before, like the works of Marquez and Hemingway. "You know how many English classes I had in college?" he laughs. "One! It was a writing class and I got a C."

Another source of satisfaction is his computer. Although he no longer works as an audio and voice-recognition software developer – a job he loved – the wired world still offers challenge and interest, particularly through chess, which he plays with people in all parts of the globe.

"There are days when I feel 'Oh man, it would be good to hack some code,'" he says with a shrug. "My company would let me work from here, but you either work or you don't. So I'm not working, and I've got to tell you, the stress relief has been just great. Why hassle with deadlines when I don't have to."

Scott feels fortunate to have this option, made possible by good financial planning during his working years. Hillary still works two half-days a week as a massage therapist, but worries about leaving Scott alone. "I can't bear to thing of him falling and not being able to get up," she explains. Although his right arm has lost all movement, and he finds walking increasingly difficult, with Hillary's help he is still able to negotiate the stairs to their bedroom. They block out an hour each morning to get Scott ready for the day, because he now needs help with showering and dressing. Sometime soon, they plan to build an extension to the house so that everything he needs is on one level.

Hillary's concern for Scott is shared by many. His family and friends have rallied to support him, visiting as often as they can. A young nephew created a beautiful and imaginative book of images, poems and thoughts for him. Eight of Scott's running mates participated in this year's Boston Marathon in his names, raising awareness of the ravages of ALS and contributing over $41,000 to research on the disease.

But it is not in Scott's nature merely to receive love and caring. His heightened perceptions have given him a fuller appreciation of the beauty in the world and the people in his life, and he continually seeks ways to give to others. One way is to be totally present for those who visit him. Another is to reach out to children. He has visited several local schools to talk to seventh graders, because he is concerned that death is a subject that is never brought out in the open.

"I start out by telling them I have a terminal disease, and I ask them if they know what that means. We get it out in the air right away. They get a firsthand view of how I'm coping with it, and that fortifies them. It might help them cope with whatever problems they have." He goes on to talk about Lou Gehrig, encouraging them to think about what someone who had played baseball for 13 years might say on retiring. "You want them to make the jump and say, 'I'm so grateful to the people who supported me so that I could do this.' And some kids do come up with that right away." He adds with a smile, "I would love to have been a teacher. I get so much enjoyment out of being with kids."

It is perhaps in his interaction with young people that his message of affirmation and strength comes across most clearly. He urges them to be more conscious of their lives, to focus on what they have rather than what they don't have, to work on their weaknesses, not bask in their strengths. He stresses how important it is to do what you love and to do it well, but to realize that you are more than your outward achievements.

In a recent talk to students at a leadership camp, Scott summarized the attitude that has enabled him to face challenges and work through problems.

"How does one deal with becoming dependent on others for life's daily activities? The simple acts of eating and bathing, impossible to do without help. What will it be like to no longer be able to say 'I love you'?

The muscles of speech too weak to function. To have the physical activities that you love so much slowly stripped away? No more putting on a pair of running shoes and going for a relaxing run.

"The answers to these questions and how we face life's adversities come from within ourselves. Throughout our lives, we are constantly learning how to adapt to the changes that are going on both internally and externally. How do we measure the success of this adaptation? Sometimes we compare ourselves to others who we think are successful. Although this is an easy thing to do, we are not being true to ourselves by making such a comparison. Each individual's success must be solely based one each individual's goals. After all, it is your life to live and no one else's...

"Earlier I told you, for the past three years I have been fighting a disease, which in all likelihood will take my life. But what I didn't tell you is, for the past three years I have been fighting a disease that will never claim my life."

By Tracy Hill

Nancy Sharon Timlin was a mother, and an inspiration. She remains her children's gift in the fight to find the cure for ALS.

She was born on August 13, 1941 in Abilene, Texas to Jake and Opal Beyer. Growing up on the Texas plains, she learned, early, the values of faith and family. The eldest daughter of six children, she was expected to be a guide and helper to her younger brothers and sisters.

She brought the same loving devotion and fierce commitment to rearing her own three daughters and one son. Her legacy lives on in the way her children each reflect her gifts and values – in Jeri Lynn, her flair for color and design; in Tracy, her creativity in art and sewing; in Sherri, her steadfast determination and lion heart; and in Mike, his discipline and passion.

How does one offer but a glimpse of her life? You are familiar with Sharon if you have felt fiercely protective of your family; if you have enjoyed watching the seasons change in New England; or if you have gotten up early, as she often did, just to watch the sunrise and revel in the glory of another day.

Sharon was a person not of likes or dislikes, but of passions: She loved curling up with a good book, creating a colorful painting, and beading costumes and wedding dresses for those she loved. She especially loved spending countless hours at the baseball field watching her son become the wonderful athlete and man he is today.

Sharon always focused on the positive in life and left the rest to prayer. In times of trial and trouble, she would say, "Don't sweat the small stuff," and soldier on.

As adults, her grown children would marvel at the wellspring of love and generosity this woman had: She took in her children's friends and every stray animal who crossed her kids' paths. She had a playful streak, too. When she was blessed with grandchildren, she nibbled the middle of the carrots on Christmas eve, so it would seem like the reindeer really had had a snack. Her grandchildren learned the wonders of nature when she would spend time with them in her garden.

She was not a traditionalist. She hewed to her own ideals. There seemed to live a gypsy in her soul.

Early in the year of 2000, she began noticing her right foot seemed to drag, but with the same determination she lived her life, she chalked it up to being in a hurry and tripping and thought nothing of it.

By the end of that same year she was walking with a cane, and everyone knew there was more to her troubles than tripping. Finally, in May of 2001, after countless doctor visits, Sharon and her family learned she had ALS. By July, Sharon was getting around by wheelchair only. Even though the disease moved quickly through her body she maintained her positive spirit.

Sharon lost her battle to the horrible disease on March 12, 2002.

We are all so grateful to have had the time with her that we did. Her courage in the face of this dreadful disease has inspired all of us to do what we can to raise awareness, contribute to research, and provide solace to those faced with ALS.

By Drew Hoffman

Sometimes in life, we are the beneficiaries of a coincidence, or a random act, or, perhaps, the moon and the stars just being in the right alignment. So it is with Clear Channel's wonderful partnership with the Angel Fund.

The catalyst in this story proved to be a simple phone call, placed by Paul DelVecchio, in 1998. Paul's wife had contracted ALS and was losing the battle.

Fueled by his determination to raise public awareness about this difficult disease, Paul grabbed the Yellow Pages and just began dialing. Fortunately for him, and for us, one of his calls was to Clear Channel Outdoor, and the person on the other end of the line was Lois Catanzaro, director of public affairs. That initial conversation has led to an alliance that today is giving hope to those battling this most difficult disease.

Between August of 1999 and April of 2004, Clear Channel has donated a total of $862,000 in billboard space to the Angel Fund. One billboard on Route 128 helped raise over $100,000 for the annual Walk of Hope, and attracted more than 1,100 participants.

Through Clear Channel Outdoor's statewide Cover Up program, the Angel Fund pays for the printing of the board, and when Clear Channel has space available, the Angel Fund's board goes up.

With the urgent need to raise awareness about the disease and the need for funding, Clear Channel is gratified to have the opportunity to give back to the community by lending their product — outdoor advertising — to such a worthy cause.

The Angel Fund is all about research, research that benefits Mass General Hospital and Dr. Bob Brown, who is one of the leading doctors in the world in ALS research. Many of the people who work or volunteer on behalf of the cause are, sadly, intimately aware of this disease: They have a relative or friend who has the disease.

The Angel Fund predicts it will raise over a million dollars this year. That is good news, but the need for funding continues. As president of Clear Channel, I know we will continue to work hand in hand with the Angel Fund to fulfill the worthy goals of this mission.

By Richard Kennedy

To tell my brother Jimmy's story and do it justice, I must begin with our father's story.

Christopher F. Kennedy was a Harvard graduate and veteran of World War II who became vice president of Northeastern University. Somewhere he found time to serve on the Quincy School Committee, and enough other volunteer committees and boards to fill the rest of this page. We eight children, however, just knew him as the perfect dad, who not only found time to help with our math homework, but also to explain the intricacies of a Major League curveball, or anything else that might have us baffled.

My dad's well-ordered life took a terrible turn after his 65th birthday and subsequent retirement from Northeastern. At his retirement party, it was noticed that his right hand had noticeably weakened, as though he'd suffered a stroke. In his typically stoic, old-school-Irish way, he had apparently ignored the weakness, and several other symptoms as well. True to his heritage, he needed to be dragged to an appointment with a neurologist.

Examination led to a CAT scan, which revealed that my dad had multiple brain tumors that seemed to explain his weakness. Surgery and subsequent radiation devastated his body, making life difficult for my mother, his primary caregiver at home. Her repeated questions to doctors were typically explained away, his steady deterioration blamed on the effects of radiation. At this point Jimmy, being the youngest child (21 years old at the time) moved in to assist my mother in caring for my dad. Cruelly, it was thus Jimmy who saw most closely the slow progress of what we later would realize was ALS.

After the official diagnosis of ALS was made, mercifully my dad didn't last much longer. On July 4, 1989, he died, leaving his family heartbroken. Despite fairly extensive research, none of us realized that there was a genetic component to ALS.

As the youngest child, Jimmy took something from each sibling in a way that made us all proud of his accomplishments. He gained notoriety in high school as an outstanding football player and track star, while excelling academically as well. He graduated with high honors from Northeastern University 11 months after my father's death, and began study at Georgetown University Law School. There, he fell in love with Washington, D.C., and began to envision a career in politics. In short order he graduated, accepted a position with a law firm, passed the bar, and proposed marriage to his girlfriend of several years, Karen Dustin. Jimmy and Karen settled in suburban Waldorf, Maryland, and appeared to have everything they had ever dreamed of.

Shortly thereafter, Jimmy began to experience weakness in his hands and legs. In keeping with the stoic Irish traditions of our father, he told no one. When he began to lose his balance with regularity, he decided that he could no longer keep things from his wife. As he prepared himself to break the news, she told him that she was pregnant. So as not to alarm Karen, Jimmy sat on his bad news for a while longer. Finally giving in to the inevitable, he was examined at Johns Hopkins Medical Center where he was given the excruciating diagnosis of ALS. He was 28 years old, and his wife was four months pregnant.

Jimmy fought a heroic three-year battle with ALS; a battle in which he never gave way to weakness, nor stopped believing he would get better, nor lost his sense of humor. His most bitter disappointment was that he was never able to hold or play with his son, Trevor. As Trevor took his first steps, Jimmy lost the ability to do the same; as Trevor began to speak, Jimmy found himself unable to respond.

Shortly after his 31st birthday, when ALS finally robbed him of his ability to breathe, Jimmy died. Like his father, Jimmy left a legacy of accomplishment and a legion of heartbroken friends.

Among those stung by Jimmy's death were two close friends of the Kennedy family, John Webb and Marty Levenson. They decided that the best way to honor the memory of such an avid runner would be to stage a road race in his name. Thus was conceived The Jimmy Kennedy Memorial Run for ALS.

Our inaugural event in June, 1998, came about through the cooperation of hundreds of dedicated volunteers. Despite a deluge of rain, and rookie race organizers, the event was an unqualified success. We were embraced by the City of Quincy and Mayor James Sheets proclaimed ALS Awareness Week in Quincy for the period preceding the second race. Event Number Three saw an ever-broadening base of volunteer support, athletes and children. We had become many things to many people: a first-class road race attracting talented runners; a family event providing carnival-like entertainment for children; a successful fund-raising vehicle benefiting ALS research; and, perhaps most significantly, a gathering spot for family and friends of ALS victims to meet, share memories, and pay tribute to loved ones.

We anticipate that all future Jimmy Kennedy Memorial Runs for ALS will be bigger and better than the earlier ones. We therefore invite all runners, all walkers, and ANYONE interested in finding a cure for ALS to join us.

By Thomas J. Kwiatkowski, Jr., M.D., Ph.D.

I stumbled on to the Angel Fund quite by accident. It was 1999 and I was finishing my residency training in neurology at the Mayo Clinic, and looking for a place to start the next phase of my career. The Angel Fund was just gathering the funds for the first Angel Fund Fellow position at Massachusetts General Hospital. I made a phone call to Dr. Robert Brown, arranged a visit to his lab in Boston, and soon I was a member of Team ALS.

I had studied for decades, literally – college, medical school and graduate school, internship, residency, fellowship. All along I knew I would eventually find a disease to study. My choices were limitless at first but, as I advanced in my training, I had to narrow my focus a little more at each stage. In my undergraduate days at Duke University, all of the sciences that dealt with human biology fascinated me – biochemistry, pharmacology, cell biology, and more.

As an M.D./Ph.D. student at Baylor College of Medicine, I was forced to select a single department in which to pursue graduate studies. I chose the newly established molecular genetics department, getting in on the ground floor of what has since developed into one of the premier genetics programs in the world. My graduate studies further focused on neurodegenerative disorders; my residency training at Mayo Clinic refined that focus to nerve and muscle diseases (both particular specialties of the Mayo Clinic).

At the same time that my brain was marching logically down the pathways of scientific endeavor, my heart was gravitating towards the patients I felt needed me most.

I had seen human suffering of all sorts, but I felt a special pull to people living with ALS, and to their families. Every story I heard unfolded with eerie similarity – the robust health and happiness encroached upon by a nagging limp or thick-tongued speech, the "tough it out" phase, the months of seeking answers...

Yet, every person had his or her own poignant twist. However, I cannot remember a single ALS patient who suffered from self-pity. It was always some variation on these consistent refrains: "I don't want to be a burden," or "What about my children?" or even "How can I help the research?"

My visit to Boston convinced me that this was where I was supposed to be. Dr. Brown told me that it would be another year before he had the funds for the position I sought. I decided to wait – I would spend a year acquiring further experience in degenerative neurological disorders, at the Mayo Clinic in Scottsdale, Arizona.

I saw patients with Alzheimer's disease, Parkinson's Disease, and every type of nerve and muscle disease, and I saw more people with ALS.

It was in Scottsdale that I met Charlotte, a delightful lady who dealt with her ALS with grace and humor. She asked if she could write to me after I left Arizona, and so she formed a bridge of sorts for me, from my training days to my Angel Fund Fellow days.

I keep her e-mails to remind me of the path I took…and the reasons why I am here. Charlotte had been a teacher, and she decided that a little trouble talking and walking was not going to take her away from her vocation, so she switched to teaching English courses on-line. Her attitude on living and dying is worth sharing: "Everyone is dying when you think of it…if you realize that your journey thru life is only so long after birth…but while one is still breathing one is ALIVE."

She was not afraid to criticize doctors who did not share her zest for living: "I really believe that subconsciously docs figure you are on your way out anyway so just sedate us and let it go. I told my primary that I'm not going any place yet – she was shocked I'd say that."

Fortunately, I shared Charlotte's view and, so, stayed on her "good doc" list.

Charlotte's letters continued in full good-cheer mode, which belied her dwindling physical condition. She continued to share stories with me, ask about my life, and inquire about ALS research, from gammaglobulin to stem cells to genetics.

The last letter I received from her ended with "What's new in Boston?"

The next letter I received began "This is Charlotte's daughter…"

I dashed off a goodbye letter that was read to her at her bedside in the hospice, which her daughter assured me Charlotte heard.

It being a final letter, I spoke in bold terms of my admiration of her and my commitment to conquering this disease: I only hope that some day soon her daughter will hear news of "what's new in Boston."

By George K. Mazareas

The last few years have been filled with many of the beautiful things fairy tales are made of: regaining vision in my eye after being blind for 25 years; marrying the woman I love in a fantasy-like wedding that took place in Greece; building and moving into our dream house; and, in the most beautiful vision of all, witnessing the birth of our baby girl whose healthy presence on earth defied all odds.

Now, looking back, I thankfully savor every moment. For the irony is this: during those happiest of times I was oblivious to the fact that ALS was quietly eating away at my body.

Suffering with ALS during the prime of my life is certainly not where I want to be. Nevertheless, like so many others, that is exactly where I am. To say I have been dealt a bad hand or thrown a curve ball is to ignore the cruel reality of ALS. It would be more accurate to say I have been thrown or dealt a death blow. These statistics don't lie. Even though there is much that is not known about ALS, the mortality rate and prognosis are well documented.

The day I learned my diagnosis might be ALS I left the doctor's office only to sit in my car and cry, for what seemed like hours. It would the first of many overwhelmingly sad moments. A few weeks later, after many more tests, I was to finally receive a definitive diagnosis. My wife, Cynthia, and I pulled into the parking garage next to my doctor's office. Even though there was an outside chance that I might not have ALS, in my gut I knew the score. I sat frozen in the passenger's seat, paralyzed by fear, shaking my head and crying uncontrollably. Cynthia held me, telling me everything would be all right.

As my doctor broke the news my wife began weeping. Strangely enough, during this ugly moment of truth, I was overcome with a surreal calm and sense of clarity.

I had, at a very early age, decided to live my life by focusing on the positive things this world had to offer, and not be weighed down the by negative elements. As a matter of fact, I have always been accused of "wearing rose-colored glasses," especially when I refused to remain upset over any situation.

Now, here I was, with my life about to undergo unimaginable changes. Reaching out, I took my wife's hand and held it tight.

During my life I have experienced many defining moments, but none like that day. On that day I refused to die with ALS. I, instead, decided to LIVE with ALS. Some could say that I have no choice in the matter, and they would be partly right. There is no cure for ALS…not even a viable therapy. Nevertheless, everyone has a choice and I have chosen to live with a purpose and a goal – to do anything and everything humanly possible to raise awareness and find a cure for ALS. Thus, I chose to get involved with the Angel Fund.

From generation to generation there is an undeniable cycle of life that goes from the cradle to the grave. With each cycle passes yet another generation and with each generation comes yet a better opportunity to find a cure. Whenever I look into my little girl's eyes I am reminded of that defining moment when I chose to live with ALS so she would never have to.

Peace, Love and Energy.

By Maureen Neil

Our family first became involved with the Angel Fund in August of 1998, following the death of my husband, Jimmie Neil, from ALS in 1997.

Since not much money goes into ALS research, the Angel Fund is critical. We had seen Ginny DelVecchio on television and I called her husband, Paul. We had several conversations about the devastation that results from this horrible disease. Following Jimmie's death, my sons, who were 14 and 12 at the time, and I went to visit them at their Winchester home and gave them some of the unused supplies that we still had – some related to the ventilator. I remember there were angels hanging everywhere. Every time I see an angel, I think of Ginny…and my husband…as well as my sister, Janet, who passed away from lung cancer at age 39 less than two years ago.

Although we did not see Dr. Robert Brown at MGH on a regular basis for care, we did see him for a second opinion in December, 1994 to confirm the ALS diagnosis of Dr. William Brown of New England Medical Center.

It took physicians two years to diagnose Jimmie with ALS. He had seen his primary care physician and was then sent to two neurologists, a neurosurgeon and an orthopedic doctor. He also had several months of physical therapy and, ultimately, even had back surgery. Although he continued to get worse, he continually kept hearing that it would take time for him to recover from the surgery, possibly up to a year.

By the time he was diagnosed, he had already gone from a cane, to a walker, to a wheelchair. The boys were only 11 and 9 at the time. In one day my four brothers-in-law built a nice wooden ramp into our house.

I'll always remember the day we were told that he would have only about three years to live – since he had already had the disease for two years at that point: It was two days before Thanksgiving. To this day I am thankful that he was in our lives.

We'd had such a good life together. We did everything with the kids – we went to Bermuda, Florida and the Cape, and took many day trips. As the ALS progressed, we still tried to do things, but it was very difficult. One night the four of us sat in the kitchen, crying, as he told us that he didn't want to leave us and still wanted to have fun. Even though he was in a wheelchair, he would still help out at the concession stand at Little League games played by our sons. He had not made the decision whether to go on a ventilator or not, but when breathing problems came very suddenly, he decided to utilize the ventilator.

After Jimmie was in the hospital for five weeks, we were finally able to take him home, just in time for Christmas of 1995. The social worker at Vencor Hospital in Boston was against it. But, finally, Jimmie became the first person that hospital had ever released to go home and be on a ventilator. The care at first was overwhelming – since he could not be left alone at all.

No one can really describe life with ALS unless you have lived it.

Several people, including my sons, Mike and Chris, were trained to do suction for him. After he was home for only about a month, we took him to the Cape for a weekend. But it turned into a disaster. Literally. It took us four hours to get there because of a huge snowstorm. And when we got there, we couldn't do anything... So, needless to say, we did not try that again.

I continued to work, so that we would be able to keep our house. And I hired an excellent person to care for him. Every Saturday I would try and take the kids somewhere. Jimmie was happy that they were able to get out, but his face looked so sad as we were leaving.

Ultimately, we had several wonderful caregivers I called upon frequently. They would try to make him laugh and took excellent care of him. Aside from them, it was very hard for us; several times a week the VNA would send a new home health aide, many of whom had no experience with a ventilator.

Jimmie said his best Father's Day was when we stayed home and watched videos together in June of 1996.

As time went on though – in spite of the fact his mind was fully in tact – he could only move his eyes to communicate with us. So, communication of any kind was very difficult. Today, there are a lot of new communication products available.

My kids were wonderful with helping with the care for their father. Michael would never complain, even though he would sometimes have to get up at 3 o'clock in the morning, on a school night, to help me. And Chris was caring for him, alone, the day before he died.

One week before Jimmie passed away, a brand new caregiver stole all our gold jewelry, including his wedding ring. He had wanted to be buried with his ring, but that became impossible.

Michael had gone on a much needed vacation with his friend's family to Baltimore on Sunday, August 17, and had to return two days later, alone, on a plane when his father died.

Some kids turn to drugs and alcohol when a major event such as a parent's death affects their lives: But Mike and Chris have honored their father's memory and have turned out to be fine young men who care about family and friends. They are now 21 and 19, and are both in college. One of Jimmie's hopes and dreams was always for them to graduate from college.

We are now planning our Seventh Annual Raffle and Softball Game between the North Cambridge Little League coaches and the Cambridge Babe Ruth League coaches to raise money for the Angel Fund. We started this to keep Jimmie alive in our hearts and minds and most people who contribute knew him very well. He was always laughing and pleasant; he would help everyone he could and I never heard him say a bad word about anyone. Each year we seem to do a little better and, last year, raised almost $4,000. Hopefully, this year will even be better.

Maybe this will also be the year that a cure for ALS will be developed through Angel Fund research.

By Derek Pearson

(Editor's note: This poem was written by David Odams's then 12-year-old nephew. David's sister and her family, including Derek, lived right next door.)

David Odams

If David Odams came back a ghost
First thing he'd do is propose a toast
Right now he is dancing in the clouds
Happy 'cause he doesn't have to wear a shroud
Everybody knows he is in heaven
Everybody knows his daughter is only seven.

David was a great athlete excelling at every sport
David was a dad who helped his sons build a fort
David loved all motorized vehicles
He actually thought they created miracles
Everybody knows he is in heaven
Everybody knows his daughter is only seven.

David taught me every day is a blessing
He taught me every lie is worth confessing
David had to leave his sons who were ten and five
Such a beautiful family all glad to be alive
Everybody knows he is in heaven
Everybody knows his daughter is only seven.

At the time I graduated from Northeastern University, with a Liberal Arts degree in June of 1971, I'm sure all I could have told you about Lou Gehrig's disease is that one of the greatest players in baseball history died of it. By the fall of 1972, when I left my reporter's job with the *Lewiston (Maine) Daily Sun* (a job I first held as a Northeastern Co-operative Education student, in the summer of 1969) to begin a master's degree at the University of Southern Maine, I'd learned first hand of its insidious and lethal nature and seen all I wanted of its devastating effects upon loved ones and friends.

While I was working as a general assignments reporter at the *Lewiston Daily Sun*, in November of 1971, the man I secretly regarded as my mentor, and the writer I hoped I would emulate as a career professional, Dick Kisonak, was diagnosed with the disease.

Dick was an engaging paradox of abilities and personality traits. Very reserved and unobtrusive to all appearances, he was a dynamic state house reporter, respected and genuinely liked by members of both sides of the aisles in the Maine Senate and the Maine House of Representatives. He found a way to be tough but fair in his dealings and writings. Though he almost never talked about it he'd been an outstanding high school baseball player who had played semi professionally. A fiercely patriotic man who served in the Navy, he went AWOL – briefly – to marry his high school sweetheart, Beverly, when he learned she was engaged to marry another.

In an article for a Portland, Maine Sunday newspaper, which subsequently went nationwide on an Associated Press news wire, Dick wrote in a chilling lead sentence: "I am scheduled to die this year." He noted: "Will I be able to die with dignity? God, I hope so…I have agreed to put my feelings down on paper…because of the possibility that what I have to say might be of some help in the future to somebody else. My message, for what it is worth, is that I have been able to adjust mentally to a point where I am able to cope so far with this awful thing that is pulling me down. Things aren't the same any more, of course, but at the same time my life is more beautiful and meaningful than ever before." In his concluding thoughts he said: "I made up my mind to live one day at a time, enjoying life to the fullest, and soon I was doing just that. A wonderful, understanding wife and children make it possible."

I was joined by a number of employees from all departments of the newspaper, and we organized a benefit softball game between the *Sun* staff and the Lewiston Police Department to help with Dick's medical costs. I treasure the card I received after the game from him, with its gently mocking "You lost!" and the clearly heartfelt expressed gratitude to all involved.

Dick lived for almost a year after I left Lewiston for graduate school and part-time work at the Portland daily newspapers. He died with the same quiet dignity he had lived, on August 7, 1973, and was mourned by an entire community. His last words to his wife, scribbled on a piece of paper, reportedly were: "Keep cool." I've always regretted I never got to say goodbye, or tell him how much I admired him.

We flash ahead now, to the fall of 1995.

I was editor of the *Winchester Town Crier*, a weekly community newspaper in the small but beautiful and affluent town of Winchester, Massachusetts, just a dozen miles northwest of Boston. A group of Winchester residents, representing a friend of theirs, was offering me "an exclusive," a chance to speak to a courageous woman battling Lou Gehrig's disease, a woman who could no longer speak but would be able to type out her answers to my questions in computer messages. I was told I was selected over the editor of the rival weekly newspaper and the editor of the Winchester edition of the regional daily newspaper because of the passion and the compassion I displayed in my writings on the editorial page.

Compliments and exclusives aside, I knew from the moment I heard the name of the disease the woman was afflicted with that I did not want to go.

Ginny DelVecchio changed all that dread in just a few moments. Nursery school administrator and teacher, artist and tennis player, wife and mother, she lived each day with a vitality many would find enviable. More than a decade before, her mother had contracted ALS. When Ginny discovered there were no services, to provide equipment or counseling for such victims, she founded the first support group for ALS in Massachusetts. Then, while providing daily care for her mother, she found herself needed to help her brother who had also contracted the deadly disease. ALS, until the last decade or so, was so rare it often took months to correctly diagnose: Ginny had the almost Herculean burden of providing daily care for two loved ones with this fatal disease, an excruciating responsibility considering the emotional, physical, psychological and, most definitely as well, financial toll ALS exacts upon victim and loved ones.

The confident, upbeat resolve Ginny adopted never, ever wavered. She became the first president of that ALS support group and continued to carry the fight, long after both her mother and brother had succumbed to the disease. She helped secure special wheelchairs, with neck braces, for victims. She helped insure an office was created, to provide equipment and information and to be a conduit for 24-hour contact with counseling professionals. "When I went looking for someone who my mother could talk to about this disease, I couldn't find anyone," she explained to me. "I didn't want others to suffer that way." She helped garner public awareness for the disease, through benefit events, and even worked with the Boston Red Sox to establish an annual Lou Gehrig's disease awareness day at Fenway Park; it was fortuitous that then Red Sox general manager James "Lou" Gorman had long arrived at his first-name nickname because of his family's affection for Lou Gehrig.

That Ginny, herself, would contract the disease made this a family tragedy of Shakespearean proportions. And the poignant irony of this lovely, vivacious woman now having to avail herself of the very life-support services she was instrumental in making possible would haunt me most every time I thought about her.

Further, I was intrigued by her unflinching, unquestioning faith ("With God, anything is possible," she was fond of saying). I was captivated by her devoted husband Paul and a coterie of gold-nugget friends like Carolyn, Sue and Jan, who cared for and playfully joked with Ginny, with equal ease.

Ultimately, I was inspired by her determined resolve to not go gently into that good night, but rather, to make herself the perfect human guinea pig that might help the renowned Dr. Robert H. Brown, Jr., of Harvard University and the research staff of Massachusetts General Hospital, to discover a cure for ALS. For Dr. Brown the research is sincerely personal: His mother died of the disease. To date, he is the only person in the world to have discovered a gene for ALS and, in fact, that gene he discovered is a familial gene, the very type present in Ginny's case but only present in about 10 percent of all ALS cases. On a personal level, I found the brilliant Dr. Brown to have an extraordinary personality – low-key, yet charismatic. We also shared a mutual love of the State of Maine and long distance running.

Finally, and most significantly, I came to understand Ginny's selfless determination to beat the disease was for her two sons' sake: Her deepest and most important resolve must be to find a cure so neither of her sons and their progeny to come would ever have to face this scourge that had so plagued her bloodline.

At about this same time syndicated *Detroit Free Press* sports writer Mitch Albom was making, as he wrote in his national best-seller **Tuesdays with Morrie**, regular trips in from Detroit and his newspaper office to the nearby Boston suburb of Waltham, to see his beloved former professor afflicted with ALS. Just a couple of communities away, I had "Wednesdays with Ginny." As soon as my newspaper went to press and my editorial responsibilities came to rest for one week's edition, around noontime on Wednesday, I would go to her house for a chat. Albom was free for his trips because his newspaper was on strike; within six months I would be completely free because my newspaper was being put to death. An "Evil Empire" of a corporation giant was at work in the greater Boston area and Eastern Massachusetts, gobbling up community newspapers as part of a shameless mega advertising pyramid, and my paper and the arch-rival *Winchester Star* were both within its sights. Within one year's time, the Fidelity-owned Community Newspaper Company had purchased both Winchester newspapers and, since the *Star* had existed since 1880 and the *Town Crier* was only two years old with a higher payroll, our paper was terminated. The final edition appeared just two weeks after I ran the 1996 Boston Marathon. Perspective made all the difference: I was losing my job; Ginny was losing her life.

At our chats I learned to wipe the spittle from her face with one smooth, matter-of-fact caring touch, and never lost my awe for the grace and dignity with which Ginny always accepted that help. I learned to carry on one-way conversation, when she lost the ability to type out extended, and then, even one-word messages. I would talk to her about everything from town happenings and events covered in that week's newspaper, to the beloved Rock 'n' Roll music of our shared Sixties generation, to my daughter's budding tennis career. Her computer was stocked with several programmed messages, to be used as responses. One comic-sad declaration was the "Damn it!" phrase, used to express frustration; another was the touching "I love you" declaration, which I was privileged to hear directed to me.

As an avid runner, with more than 25 marathons completed, I often talked to Ginny about how my training was going for that spring's special edition of the Boston Marathon, the 100th anniversary run. It was then that I suggested to Ginny and Paul that I would like to run the 1996 Boston Marathon to honor Ginny and her battle with ALS, and that per-haps the three of us could create an ALS fund to be solely a research fund, supporting the work of Dr. Brown. Ginny's response was that stunning warm smile of hers…and a "thumbs up" signal. We were on our way.

Vividly, however, I remember how horrified I was when I learned Ginny wanted to attend the massive pasta feed the Boston Marathon organizers host for entrants and their loved ones, just prior to the running of the marathon. How could poor Ginny want to attend that? How could she want to be surrounded by thousands of people, with fit and vibrant bodies that allowed them, indeed, in Thoreau's words, to "suck the marrow out of life," and live life for its ultimate vitality…while she sat strapped to a chair, stripped of all control and use of her body? How could she want to be surrounded by thousands who ate and thoroughly enjoyed a wonderful meal…while she took nourishment through a feeding tube? Yet, Ginny simply glowed that evening. A number of athletes, completely unknown to any of us, stopped by our table, merely to offer a friendly word and, ultimately, their support. Some even asked to see how her computer worked. I would later reflect that Ginny wasn't a jealous or bitter person, so the experience wasn't at all painful; she simply wanted to be back among those who lived life to its fullest, and this opportunity thrilled her. I had to be one of the proudest runners in the World Trade Center in Boston that night: Ginny was my guest…and I had helped her to "escape" ever so briefly the nightmare of the captivity ALS presented to her at home.

Thus, I ran and was very fortunate to finish the 1996 Boston Marathon for Ginny. I had injured my right foot in training about 10 days before the marathon, and icing and Advil tablets were insuring only that I could start the event. Gone were any hopes that I could do an "easy" three and one-half hour run, or less, and not force Ginny to wait an extended time for me to finish. Indeed, it was only when I reached Kenmore Square, less than one mile from the finish and barely under four hours, that I finally KNEW my body would allow me to finish…even if I had to walk. And, ultimately, I was privileged to present her with my special gold-plated finisher's medallion in the VIP tent, just beyond the finish line in Boston's Copley Square. We promoted the Ginny DelVecchio Fund as best we could. I had unabashedly run news accounts and used editorial space in my newspaper, and we wallpapered Winchester with flyers about our cause. Ultimately, the fund did so well that Dr. Brown drew from its account more than $400,000 to purchase a new DNA imaging machine for his research lab.

What followed were more events to help fortify Ginny's will to continue her fight and to continue to support the research fund. I ran the Boston Marathon again in her honor in 1997 and then, as a Mother's Day gift to Ginny, on the week of May 12-18, 1997, I did a statewide run of Massachusetts, running west to east, 162 miles in seven days. We received wonderful support from the Winchester community to defray costs. The run went beautifully, concluding with me pushing Ginny across a ceremonial finish line in front of St. Mary's Church in Winchester, before a large group of loved ones, friends and St. Mary's parishioners. A documentary film about my relationship with Ginny and the statewide run was made by MediaOne and played on several community channels around the Boston area, further helping to boost awareness and support the fund. Then, again in 1998, I ran the Boston Marathon to continue the momentum.

But, sadly, the dying of the light was coming for Ginny. After the 1998 Boston Marathon I found myself at a complete loss about what came next. A cure no longer seemed possible soon enough for her. Clearly, the three-year fight was taking its toll on her, her family, her friends. She had dissipated to the point she was on life-support systems for breathing, for taking in nourishment, and for voiding wastes. Ginny made a decision: She had had enough, and she chose a specific day to shut off all life-support systems.

Paul, her family, and her friends called me in Maine, the day before, to say goodbye. I was trembling as I told her how inspirational she would always be to me, and that the fight to find a cure would continue. Then I suddenly heard myself saying: "I'll be running the Boston Marathon this coming spring, and this time you'll be able to watch me and be with me all the way."

Clearly, in the background, I heard Ginny's computer for the last time: "I love you."

Ginny DelVecchio died on August 10, 1998, just three days after the 25th anniversary of Dick Kisonak's death. I ran the 1999 Boston Marathon, and I'll always believe Ginny was there too.

Today, the Ginny DelVecchio Fund has evolved into the Angel Fund, embraced by others fervently hoping to find a cure for ALS. In 2001, to celebrate the 35th anniversary of the day she became the first woman ever to run and complete the Boston Marathon, Roberta "Bobbi" Gibb honored me with an invitation to run with her at Boston. And, because she had a friend battling ALS, she, too, joined the cause of those running Boston in support of the Angel Fund.

Bobbi, who grew up in Winchester, was still a resident of the town when she stunned organizers of the Boston Marathon by running it with the 400-to-500 men present in 1966. She was someone I first met in 1996 when, as editor of the *Winchester Town Crier*, I was looking for a significant Winchester connection to the marathon and its 100th anniversary celebration. I did the story and we subsequently became friends. I told her my very first newspaper column, written as a freshman at Northeastern University in the spring of 1967, was about how women should be allowed to run the Boston Marathon. I even gave her a copy of it to read, in spite of how embarrassing the unsophisticated, early attempt at column-writing proved to be. And now, it is so wonderful to have Bobbi Gibb, lending her celebrity and her integrity to the cause of the Angel Fund. Ginny would have just loved this woman!

I was deeply honored when Ginny's family made me the last speaker at her special memorial service in 1998. The beautiful and cavernous St. Mary's Church was packed with loved ones, family and friends, and many more people paying their last respects from the community of Winchester and well beyond its boundaries.

My role was then, as it must be with this very essay, to conclude with this pledge: Ginny, we best honor your courage and your memory by insuring this fight continues…until no one, ever again, has to suffer with and die of ALS. On that day, I imagine, an Angel named Ginny will smile her best sunrise stunner of a smile…and give us all a BIG "Thumbs Up."

By Debra E. Rohan

In "Musee' de Beaus Artes," W. H. Auden expresses the view that:"While someone is suffering, the world goes on, and most people go about their business without worrying too much about it."

The world does go on; however,

while someone suffers there are those out there that feel it, are moved by it, and are inspired to develop a cure and overcome the suffering. There are many people with positive "I can do it" attitudes that never give up and put forth their best effort to make a difference for the love of someone they see suffering.

It was 1976, the Bicentennial year. I was 17 and in my first year of college. That year my mom was diagnosed with ALS, or Lou Gehrig's disease. She knew for some time before that there was a problem. But now, seeing her walking with a cane, and having watched as she went through so many hospital tests, we finally understood why her speech had become slurred and why her left side was paralyzed. She was too young – she was only 56 years old.

At this time I remained true to my ways as a tomboy, spending many hours in the woods riding my pony. In school I was so shy it would make me angry with myself. I wanted desperately to get over my shyness so I entered a beauty pageant at the Liberty Tree Mall that put me in the running for the Ms. Massachusetts state pageant. I remember doing really well and won runner-up. I was so proud of myself, succeeding in spite of the fact my knees were knocking on stage as I answered the questions. I did exactly what I wanted that day – overcame my shyness.

Yet, in my glory, up on the stage, I remember looking out into the audience. I remember seeing how sad my mom looked. She was scared about her own fate, feeling so sad knowing her future with this illness might not have a happy outcome. There really wasn't much chance to discuss my winning; our concentration was on my mom as she went through times of being scared, angry and very depressed.

I felt so much sadness for her. There was no doubting that. But I also had to go on with my life. If I let them, these circumstances gave me headaches and brought me down. I remember when I was spoon-feeding her, how her mouth would clamp down on the metal spoon breaking her teeth. Eventually we had to make the decision to have a feeding tube put in to feed her. We had to make many of these unfortunate decisions as the disease progressed.

Making every effort to help her get the help she needed, my dad had taken mom to Mass General Hospital for tests, and then we went out of state to get a second opinion. While we were in Tallahassee, Florida, I met my future husband. He did her MRI and CAT scans at Tallahassee Memorial Hospital.

While we were in Florida I remember taking my mom shopping for new shoes because her left foot was starting to drag. We were looking for shoes that would make walking a little easier. I'll never forget the saleswoman whispering to me that "she must be drunk." It was painful to see how she was viewed about her speech, when her speech sometimes would get slurred and all she was trying to do was carry on with her day-to-day life. I told the saleswoman my mom did not drink.

My family, which included seven kids, alternated taking turns feeding her with a tube each meal. We would sit up with her giving my dad, regular daily breaks, over the course of 18 years. During that time her strength periodically worsened; ultimately she wound up in a wheelchair and lost the use of her voice. She was fortunate – I guess you could call it that – to have outlived the prevailing three-to-five-year statistics for ALS victims and go on for 18 years. Was it all the experimental drugs? Her religious beliefs? The abundance of love and care from my father and her children? A combination of them all? We may never know. It feels good that we tried our best.

My dad proved his genius by designing a computer system, with a sensor device, that attached to mom's glasses. This allowed her to blink her eyes to communicate through a computer. This was 25 years ago, well before computers had the capabilities they have today. Her body deteriorated, but her mind stayed sharp because of that computer. She read three or four newspapers a day, blinking her eyes for us to turn the page, and even wrote our annual Christmas letters. She also enjoyed watching the news, "Jeopardy" and "Wheel of Fortune," while my father snored, exhausted, in his recliner chair.

My dad was always trying to brighten her spirits by decorating our large two-story house, on Central Street, especially around Halloween and Christmas. He made sure she could see the lights and hear the music from their bedroom windows. The decorations blinked and twinkled all around the porch that wrapped around those windows. While brightening my mom's spirits and, hopefully, providing her spiritual hope on Christmas, and making her laugh on Halloween, my dad was also growing popular with the Town of Saugus for his decorating skills during the holidays.

As you go forth on each day, you meet new people…and special ones touch your life. I will forever be grateful to Dr. Helen Powers, one of my teachers at Marian Court College. She suggested I take my mom to a prayer meeting with Father McDonough at a church in Boston when my mom was first stricken with ALS. This was a very stressful time during my first year at Marian Court.

I will never forget the blessed event that occurred while we were at that church, singing. A white dove flew in the window and perched on the front altar. During the time my mom was first diagnosed, as I mentioned earlier, she was scared and depressed. The sudden appearance of the dove, however, brought her so much hope and gave her the power to go on. The dove's appearance at the church also deeply affected other members of my family, especially my father who continued to bring my mom to the weekly prayer meetings at that church. We believe she continued to get a spiritual lift that carried her for quite some time; she lived considerably longer than the norm for this disease, dying at the age of 73.

Over the years I married, had a family, and moved away. I always came home on every vacation to help the family out. I would scrub and clean my parents' house, and spend hours, with my children by my side, picking the wild flowers by the pond to decorate the house. I would try to make up for lost time, living so many miles away. I remember so vividly the many conversations I wanted to have but was forced to miss, with mom, when I had my children. She couldn't converse with me, when I knew I needed her for emotional support, while I was raising my young children. I felt like I really missed out on a lot then, by not having her parenting advice.

My dad passed away just a couple of years ago, after suffering congestive heart failure. That, too, was a very sad thing to watch and attempt to support him. Worse than that, though, were the three years we spent trying to treat this beautiful man's depression, taking him to mental facilities to regulate his medicine. There were other great people in this facility, individuals who were once wonderfully intelligent, like doctors and teachers, who also were afflicted with mental deterioration. Now they had to be cared for by others, so they would not hurt themselves. The suffering was so sad. And the suffering was everywhere. It reminded me, again, of that verse by Auden:

"While someone is suffering, the world goes on, and most people go about their business without worrying too much about it."

By Ron Sanders

The first indications of the disease that I recall was when my mother, Kay Sanders, was on a chair working and her leg gave out, causing her to fall. She described it as being strange that, without warning, her leg just stopped supporting her.

Some time after that I was asked to take her into Mass General Hospital for tests and I remember that day for two reasons. As I was waiting in a long, deserted hallway, an older woman came out of a door and was walking towards me. As she passed, I looked up and was surprised that it was Katherine Hepburn…and I couldn't wait to tell my mother who I saw. When my mother was finished with the exam and tests, I told her about it and she was excited too, since this lady was one of her favorite actresses. But then there was the Bad News: The doctor thought she might have MS…or it could even be a worse disease, ALS. She should hope it wasn't that one.

But it was.

I was living in Florida when I received a call at work, from back home in Massachusetts. The news was awful; her doctor projected that she had four months to two years to live. It is amazing that my mother was able to fight the disease for another 16-to-17 years after that diagnosis!

My mother wrote via computer with a system of slightly moving her hand that interrupted a light, to spell each word. With a minute or two of concentration for a single letter, she would write notes to us. Sometimes she would work for hours…only to lose the entire message through one wrong stroke. Once she wrote that the worst thing for her was the inability to fully control her emotions. She was a very stoic person and did not like to show her emotions.

It is absolutely amazing that even after almost two decades of suffering she, virtually always, had a smile when one of us came to see her.

Late in the illness I would have dreams that she would be walking and talking like anyone else, and I was able to have a conversation with her again. These were good dreams. She said that some days the symptoms went away for a while and, in her stoic way, just acted like this was part of the plan – you get the good with the bad.

We took turns at night, feeding and caring for her, and one night, in the final years, as she was watching her favorite television show, "Wheel of Fortune," I asked her to blink her eyes when she knew the answer. She did, again and again, and usually had the answer before I did. I was affected by the thought that, although she was no longer able to communicate through the computer, her mind was still doing well…but was trapped inside.

I felt guilty for not doing more of this to communicate with her, since it was obvious that she appreciated the chance to do something that would be a simple thing for others.

Through all of the pain and suffering one thing was certain: She never lost her faith. There was no question that the faith that made her drag as many of her seven children as she could to church every Sunday was just as strong right up until her last day with us.

By Irene Scaturro

In August of 1984, the lives of all the members of my family changed forever.

Later, I would come to realize that we had been building up to this point for months. All spring my husband, Frank, had been exhausted. We had chalked it up to stress, to the long days associated with starting up our new business, a gourmet and catering shop. The shop had been a dream of my husband, who had been a high school teacher.

In early summer of 1984, we began to consider that something more serious was going on with him. We had taken a Memorial Day week-end trip to the Cape to re-energize. Frank, who loved to walk on the beach, simply could not. He explained that it felt as if he were wearing lead boots. Shortly after that he started slurring his words, and his mouth seemed to droop. One of our customers, calling in an order, accused Frank of being drunk, and hung up the phone on him. We couldn't ignore the symptoms any longer.

I suspected a stroke. Our family doctor suggested we consult a neurologist after Frank's exam turned up nothing conclusive. Maybe, we should have known: Frank's mother had been diagnosed with ALS about one-to-two years before. Still, his symptoms – fatigue, and difficulty with walking and swallowing – were not her symptoms. The Massachusetts General Hospital team of doctors gave us the tragic diagnosis, of ALS, on the eve of our 20th wedding anniversary.

My mother-in-law, at the age of 69, was the first known person in her family with the disease. My husband was only 49. Not only were the symptoms of my mother-in-law different from his, the progression of the disease was very different too. With Frank, every muscle in his body seemed to be attacked simultaneously, impairing all his abilities; his mother's progression had started with her leg muscles, then gradually worked its way up her body.

All of a sudden, there was no future. There would be no growing old together. He would not see our teen-age children reach adulthood…get married…have children. Nor would we see our fledgling business flourish. I worked hours just as long, and supported the business fully – but Frank was the heart and soul of it.

What an especially cruel disease is ALS! Frank said he felt like a prisoner in his own body. His condition deteriorated quickly. Within weeks he couldn't walk, and could barely make himself understood. In spite of all this he continued teaching part-time at a local Catholic high school, and working at the business after school. I don't know how he was able to teach technical drawing to high school students for as long as he did; his spirit was strong. He managed until the Thanksgiving recess.

I could no longer put my energies into the business because Frank's condition deteriorated so quickly, and he was my top priority. I closed the doors of our business in early December of 1984, 14 months after we had first opened them together.

I was totally consumed by his care. He now needed everything done for him.

During this nightmarish time, our children suffered. They suffered because adolescence and the teen-age years are a time of inherent struggles – the struggle to fit in, the struggle to not be different. But they were different. The father they loved was dying.

Our oldest child, 18-year-old Julie, dropped out of her first year of college. She said she wanted to help with the business, even though both her father and I wanted her to stay in school. I think she was, quite simply, overwhelmed and unable to concentrate.

Steve, our 15-year-old middle child, who was usually mild-mannered and affable, became rebellious and argumentative. As the older of our two sons, he felt a responsibility we didn't want him to assume. This caused much conflict between him and his younger brother. During the first year he helped in whatever way he could. As time passed he avoided helping, more and more.

Mark was 12 years old at the time, a sensitive, compassionate child. I never had time to feel guilty while I was caring for Frank, but later, when I had time to reflect, I thought of all the times Mark should have been with his friends. Yet, he insisted on staying home. I thought of all the times he, or his brother, helped me lift their father from the wheelchair to the bed...and I'd cry.

We all struggled to survive, each in our own way. I forced myself to fully live in the present, concentrating on one day at a time or, on some days, one hour at a time. My world revolved around taking care of the basic needs of my family.

I felt blessed because there was a loving, extended family, good friends, and a lot of community support. In spite of this it became a lonely, exhausting struggle. At first, I resisted having someone in to help me, because I wanted to give my family some measure of privacy. Eventually, I needed help, just so I could recover some of my energy.

We started with several hours a week of Home Health Aid help and, during the last months of Frank's life, Hospice nurses were there all the time, which allowed me to get some sleep at night…

Months after our long battle with ALS ended, I joined my sister-in-law, Ginny DelVecchio, as she started an ALS Support Group in the Burlington/Woburn, Massachusetts area.

Throughout my husband's illness, I had become an advocate for him. So much of what I had to do was learn-as-you-go. Ginny also knew how important it was to have support, to share information and experiences. She knew how important it was just to talk about what was happening. She was the inspiration and the force behind this ALS Support Group and, later, because of her initiative and leadership the Massachusetts Chapter of the ALS Association was born.

Several years afterward, I was devastated as I took a phone call from Ginny. Devastated because of how she sounded. Her voice had that same nasal quality that my husband, Ginny's brother, had when he began his downward spiral with ALS. At that time I agreed with her – it was probably just a cold; but I felt otherwise. My fears were confirmed. Soon. She had ALS.

Ginny was a special person who gave us so much of herself throughout the course of her illness. One of the most wonderful accomplishments to come out of all Ginny's and her husband Paul's struggles was their establishment of the Angel Fund at Massachusetts General Hospital, which is devoted entirely to ALS research.

All of my children have grown to adulthood. They are kind, loving people. All of them carry scars. They lost a father, a grandmother, and a beloved aunt to a terrible disease, leaving an unspoken threat over them… and a great fear in me. One of my most fervent hopes and prayers is a cure for ALS. I dream of this happening in the near future, and so I can finally feel the burden of worry and fear being lifted from my shoulders.

This is one change in my life to which I look forward…with every fiber of my being.

By Jane Schulte

I lost one of my best friends, Sharon Timlin, to ALS. Sharon and I worked together but we were more than co-workers. I remember Sharon as being not only very knowledgeable and efficient but she could also make work fun. She was quite a character around the office -keeping us in stitches and always being so upbeat with witty sayings all the time; and always so upbeat with her attitude.

One incident in particular sticks in my mind. She had a habit of taking off her shoes and walking around the office barefooted. That drove the manager nuts and he asked her not to go around without shoes because she might step on a staple or something. So the next week Sharon showed up at the office in a pair of fuzzy "bear" house shoes. She was doing what he asked of her but she was still "bearfooted." I do believe she wore those house shoes until they were worn out.

We were very different. Sharon was Catholic and I was Methodist. Sharon preferred country music and I preferred hard rock. Sharon could grow anything and I could kill any plant that got close to me. Sharon liked cats and I liked dogs. Sharon was a 'pink' person and I was a 'blue' person. But despite all these differences, we became fast friends. We went to lunch together, talked about our families, went on trips together, etc.

I continue to miss her to this day. We sat out at the local minor league baseball games watching the games and talking. A small part of her remains close to me over the mantel in my living room. It is her first "commissioned" work of art. Sharon took up painting after her children left home and even took a course at the local junior college. I love anything Southwestern so she painted a picture of the Taos Pueblo just for me and I still treasure it.

I remember one of her favorite sayings: "When God closes a door, He opens a window." Unfortunately God has closed the door on my friendship with Sharon by taking her to be with Him. But He has opened a window for me to be able to help others with ALS by helping through the Angel Fund. Participating in the memorial 5K road race in her name has made me realize that God does have a purpose for me in life, to help others, just as Sharon always did.

By Jan Serieka

Ode to Ginny

Ginny, an angel, a mother, a friend
An inspiration of courage to the very end,
Her mother and brother had, too, this disease,
So the ALS chapter she started, to ease
The pain and suffering of all who were hit,
The flames of hope were increasingly lit.
But Lou Gehrig's disease, the foe she faced
Attacked her muscles and motion erased.
Her limbs, mouth, and tongue unable to move,
Her skills with a computer had to improve.
Determination and will dug right in
With practice and patience she began again.
With only thumb, then the twitch of a knee
She communicated and laughed with friends and fam'ly.
She fought her fight with her head held high
To help doctors' research she was willing to try
Any experimental drug, new treatment or tool
To find a real cure, this lady did rule.
Although her was poked and with a tube was fed
Ginny never lost her spirit…instead…
With deep faith and love, her heart was full
Said, "With God, nothing was impossible."
The monster won and defeated her,
Those last days passed in such a blur.
Ginny's now gone on to a better place
With peace and light and filled with grace.
But, her cause lives on – to find a cure,
That's the goal of the Angel Fund for sure.
In memory of her, we pray, walk and run
To beat ALS – we'll not stop till we're done.

By H. S. Sherrill

In the fall of 1997, before my health debacle, my friend Emily DiMaggio had suggested I help her establish the Friends of the Angel Fund with the famous Red Sox hero, Ted Williams. He and I spoke on the telephone several times in our efforts to create this separate board to support the Angel Fund. Mr. Williams sounded just like I imagined John Wayne would on the telephone! Every time I spoke with him my excitement was simply over-the-top!

At one point I was even invited to visit Ted Williams and Yogi Berra in Florida. Unfortunately, I was unable to catch my flight because my connecting flight was placed in a holding pattern between Washington and Philadelphia. I will always mourn that missed opportunity. I wanted to meet the man who said, "It ain't over…until it's over."

Emily introduced me to Paul DelVecchio, the executive director of the Angel Fund, over the telephone. Paul's personal experiences with ALS, because of his wife Ginny, were very compelling. His tale of multiple family deaths was heart-breaking. The efforts that Paul has made in association with the Angel Fund, to raise funds for research, have been extraordinary.

Thus, after I survived my illness, I felt a deep connection with those who have died from complete paralysis, through this insidious tragedy known as ALS.

You see, in February of 1998, I became partially paralyzed. The tortuous experience lingered for seven months with daily physical therapy to gain the use of my arm, to reinvigorate my shoulders, which had atrophied to just bone. My left leg went through continuously jolting nerve spasms. To this day, I suffer from numbness, pain and less energy.

Here is my story…

I was coming home from a business trip when my shoulders and back began to ache painfully. I could not get comfortable on the small plane seat. Even after I consumed a cocktail and an aspirin there was no effect. After landing at Logan Airport, I felt like the worst flu was overtaking me. In great pain I drove home, through a rainy drizzle and endless traffic, where I crawled into bed to take a nap. The pain was incredible; the aches were so strong my brain ran feverously.

I awoke several hours later and my arm hung limply from my shoulder; I could not move my arm but my hand worked. I was astonished, shocked and amazed by this overwhelming change of circumstances. I felt like my reality was slipping away from me. The searing pain ran up my back, across my shoulders and shoulder blades. My neck burned with stiffness and tension. My leg twitched with electrical tremors. The pain never went away; minute after minute the burden hung over me.

In my search to find out why this was happening to me, I visited the best doctors at the best hospitals, all of whom seemed clueless and unsupportive. One doctor even suggested placing a pin in my shoulder and upper arm to keep it permanently elevated! One neurologist thought I might have ALS. The idea that I might have ALS terrified me; my mind ran wild with the stories I had listened to only months before.

Trip after trip to the hospital, meeting with different doctors finally provided the consensus that my painful paralysis came from nerve damage across my shoulders and down my left side. I was given anti-inflammatory medicine for a month, and prescribed large doses of Motrin and a medicine to preserve the integrity of my stomach. The excruciating, throbbing pain persisted. My mind was delirious. I moved into the guest room because I could only sleep for minutes at a time. Only the cold packs and heat therapy reduced the pain. This process was repeated on the hour, twenty-four hours a day, for the months ahead. I felt like I was struggling for my life.

Contrary the beliefs of the doctors, my physical therapist Tom, at Gordon College, believed that I could rebuild the nerves. Through exertion underwater, hands on physical pressure exercise, Tom forced me to attempt to move my shoulder, arm and left leg. My progress was so slow; I felt heart-broken, my depression was so profound that my only relief was to sob endlessly, almost hysterically. It is ignorance that makes us assume so much about our health.

Tom was right! Finally, there was enough progress to kindle some faith that I might be well some day. After five months the pain slowly subsided, and the nerves were slowly reclaimed. It was a personal and emotional triumph. It changed the way I think, and it dramatically enlarged my empathy for others in need.

At the end, the doctors thought my illness was caused by Fifth's Disease, which I caught from two of my children. When children catch the disease, which is in the measles, mumps and chicken pox family, they get tired, they ache, and they get small red bumps on their flesh. Adults can suffer a broader range of pain, including paralysis and death. Without the kindness of my physical therapist Tom, and his other patients, I would not have made it through my personal ordeal.

My friends at the Angel Fund are all loving, kindred spirits who have met the human loss of family and friends. Their courage and thought-fulness have surpassed the wreckage of this tragic disease, so they can help others. Their goal is to find the cure that can ameliorate the pain and suffer-ing, and perhaps one day, through advanced research, find a cure. This path may be long, but the heart and soul of the survivors and those living today with this disease shine a great light on those that hear our cry.

By Mike Timlin

(Editor's note: For the past few seasons in every game Mike Timlin has made an appearance on the pitching mound for the Boston Red Sox, he has made a generous donations to the Angel Fund.)

This year was one of the most exciting in the history of Red Sox nation. It was a season I was honored to share with the fans, my teammates, and most importantly, my family.

As I reflect on the season, I think about the joy the game brought to my mother, Sharon Timlin, and the excitement and pride she would have felt, not only for me, but also for the whole Red Sox family. Unfortunately, my mother fought her own battle, a battle with ALS. She died of this devastating disease in 2002.

There are currently over 30,000 people in the United States who have this neuro-degenerative disease that attacks nerve cells in the brain and spinal cord and eventually muscles throughout the body. ALS does not discriminate; it knows no age limits. And there is no cure – yet.

Like many of you who have been personally affected by ALS, I am committed to finding a cure. The ALS Genetics Laboratory at Massachusetts General Hospital, run by Dr. Robert H. Brown, Jr., offers the best hope yet for a cure. The Angel Fund recently purchased a major fluid-handling robot central to the activity of the Cecil B. Day Lab at Massachusetts, under Dr. Brown. This is a major step, but more needs to be done.

That's why I am working with the Angel Fund to provide funding for the most technologically advanced equipment available to researchers. It's the path I see to "striking out" ALS.

By Mark Zullo

On December 7, 2000, my older brother David's 50th birthday, my mother, Marilyn V. Zullo, died from ALS, after a three-year struggle with this terrible disease. Her death occurred just a few days before I was to visit her in North Carolina. Her condition had been deteriorating steadily, so I expected this visit to be the last time I would see her alive…the last time I would talk to her and hug her…the last time I would be able to tell her that I loved her. But she didn't last that long and, boy, did I have regrets that I didn't have an opportunity to spend a little more time with her before she passed on at the too-young age of 70.

Over the next few months, as I was training for the 2001 Boston Marathon, I experienced those thoughts of regret often as I logged the miles necessary to complete my first marathon. However, at the same time, as I pushed and cajoled myself on those long runs (I talked to her on those runs and wondered if she could hear me…I felt she did, but…), I knew she was there too, an angel on my shoulder, helping me with each stride. So, when I reached the Marathon finish line in 3:56 (under my goal of 4 hours!), I smiled and knew she was there with me.

But then there was a letdown after the marathon (there has to be a post first marathon depressive syndrome!). I had lost one of my main coping mechanisms to deal with my loss and I was floundering a bit. Then I came across a race application for Squirrel Run IV, a race in memory of Jimmy Kennedy to benefit ALS research at Mass General Hospital. It seemed like a logical race to enter. I didn't have a good day running-wise, but I met Ratt Kennedy and the late Scott Carlson (a fellow surfer!), and I learned about the Angel Fund. It was a great event, and I knew I wanted to run the race again. Little did I realize how much the Angel Fund would become part of my life.

Fast forward to June, 2002 and Squirrel Run V. My father came up from North Carolina to present the Marilyn V. Zullo Memorial Trophy, which that year went to the second overall women's finisher. It was a special moment. After that event I continued to communicate with the Angel Fund, and learned about Team ALS, a group of runners competing in the Boston Marathon to raise money for the Angel Fund. Could this be my "in" to running Boston again? Only this time I wanted to run with my daughters Jessica, who had run one previous marathon, and Courtney, who had never run a marathon, dedicating our efforts to the memory of Mom/ Nana. Unfortunately, none of us were fast enough to be official qualifiers. But thanks to Rich Kennedy and some finagling on my part, we were able to procure three non-qualifier's numbers. So, through the nasty winter of

2002-2003, my daughters and I trained; we did all our long runs together and raised money for the Angel Fund. Once again, my mother, their Nana, was with us. We ran the 26.2 miles together, crossing the finish line with our hands clasped together, raised to the sky in jubilation. And more importantly, we raised over $10,000 for the Angel Fund!

It was a special honor to learn that, in June of 2003, at Squirrel Run VI, the Marilyn V. Zullo Trophy was now going to be awarded to the first female walker (my Mom had been an avid walker/hiker). In another special moment, the winner was my wife Dot! She has since gone on to win the award at the 2004 and 2005 Squirrel Runs as well, making our annual sojourn to Quincy a memorable day each time. In reality though, all of the Angel Fund events my family has been involved with are memorable, thanks to our friends at the Angel Fund, and the knowledge we are helping to find a cure for this devastating disease.

Over the last four and one-half years, I've often wondered what I would have said to my Mom if I had seen her that one last time…or wondered how she might have guided me had she not contracted ALS…if only she could hear me. But I know she has heard me — she helped my family find the Angel Fund, and I know a special angel is with me each time I reach into my pocket and touch the Angel Fund coin I always carry with me. We all miss you, Mom…we'll always keep your voice in our hearts.

9148662R1

Made in the USA
Lexington, KY
01 April 2011